C000104527

MANUAL OF INFECTION CONTROL
PROCEDURES

To my wife Laila, and my children Numair and Namiz for their abiding love, understanding and encouragement

MANUAL OF INFECTION CONTROL PROCEDURES

Dr. N. N. DAMANI

MSc (Lond.), MBBS, FRCPath.
Consultant Microbiologist & Infection Control Doctor
Craigavon Area Hospital Group Trust, Portadown, U.K.

Foreword by

Professor G.A.J. Ayliffe

BSc, MD, FRCPath.
Emeritus Professor of Medical Microbiology, University of Birmingham,
formerly Director of the Hospital Infection Research Laboratory, Birmingham, U.K.,
ex-Chairman of the International Federation of Infection Control.

GMM

© 1997
Greenwich Medical Media Ltd.
219 The Linen Hall
162-168 Regent Street
London
W1R 5TB

ISBN 1 900151 286

First Published 1997

While the advice and information in this book is believed to be true and accurate, neither the author nor the publisher can accept any legal responsibility or liability for any loss or damage arising from actions or decisions based in this book. The ultimate responsibility for the treatment of patients and the interpretation lies with the medical practitioner. The opinions expressed are those of the author and the inclusion in this book relating to a particular product, method or technique does not amount to an endorsement of its value or quality, or of the claims made of it by its manufacture.Every effort has been made to check drug dosages; however, it is still possible that errors have occured. Furthermore, dosage schedules are constantly being revised and new side effects recognised. For these reasons, the medical practitioner is strongly urged to consult the drug companies' printed instructions before administering any of the drugs recommended in this book.

Apart from any fair dealing for the purposes of research or private study, or criticism or review, as permitted under the UK Copyright Designs and Patents Act, 1988, this publication may not be reproduced, stored, or transmitted, in any form or by any means, without the prior permission in writing of the publishers, or in the case of reprographic reproduction only in accordance with the terms of the licences issued by the Copyright Licensing Agency in the UK, or in accordance with the terms of the licences issued by the appropriate Reproduction Rights Organization outside the UK. Enquiries concerning reproduction outside the terms stated here should be sent to the publishers at the London address printed above.

The right of Dr N.N. Damani to be identified as the author of this work has been asserted by him in accordance with the Copyright, Designs and Patents Act 1988.

The publisher makes no representation, express or implied, with regard to the accuracy of the information contained in this book and cannot accept any legal responsibility or liability for any errors or omissions that may be made.

A catalogue record for this book is available from the British Library

Distributed worldwide by
Oxford University Press

Project Manager
Gavin Smith

Production and Design by
Derek Virtue, DataNet

Printed in Great Britain

What, will these hands ne'er be clean?

WILLIAM SHAKESPEARE
Macbeth

FOREWORD

Hospital-acquired (nosocomial) infection is a major problem in the hospitals of most countries and despite improvements in control methods, the prevalence of infection remains at 5-10%. Infections are mainly of surgical wounds, the respiratory and urinary tracts, and the skin. The important risk factors for the acquisition of infection are invasive procedures which include operative surgery, intravascular and urinary catheterization and mechanical ventilation of the respiratory tract. Other risk factors include traumatic injuries, burns, age (elderly and neonates), immuno-suppression and existing disease.

Many infections are endogenous (ie, acquired from the patient's own microbial flora) and are not necessarily preventable, although infection can be kept to a minimum by good aseptic techniques. The spread of infection from patient to patient is often difficult to prevent, particularly in overcrowded hospitals with staff shortages and limited facilities. The prevention of cross-infection with highly antibiotic-resistant organisms, such as epidemic methicillin-resistant *Staphylococcus aureus* (MRSA) can be difficult and often requires considerable resources. Vancomycin-resistant enterococcal infections may be untreatable with currently available antibiotics and Gram-negative bacilli resistant to the quinolones and the third generation cephalosporins frequently cause therapeutic problems. Cross-infection can be considerably reduced by a few basic measures, for example handwashing or disinfection correctly performed at the right time. Handwashing is generally considered to be the most important single measure in infection control and is dealt with in detail in this manual. Although prevention of transmission is of major importance, the rational use of antibiotics and restriction of certain agents is necessary to achieve a long-term effect. Other organisms which have emerged in hospitals in recent years include *Clostridium difficile*, causing outbreaks in the elderly, and legionella associated with cooling towers and contaminated water supplies. Food poisoning is mainly a problem in the community, but epidemics occur in hospitals. *Escherichia coli* 0157:H7 has recently been responsible for large outbreaks of severe gastroenteritis and occasional deaths from renal failure.

The potential hazards of blood-borne viruses (hepatitis B (HBV) and C (HCV) and human immunodeficiency virus (HIV)), particularly from injuries due to sharp instruments, cause considerable anxiety to staff. Policies for the safe disposal of clinical waste, especially needles, must be correctly implemented. Spread of these blood-borne infections to patients from contaminated medical equipment is also a potential hazard and the production of safe decontamination policies is a major responsibility of infection control teams. Although decontamination of equipment by heat is the optimal method, many items are heat-labile and chemical disinfection is required. Flexible endoscopes fall into this category and are difficult to clean and disinfect. The nature of surgery is also changing and minimal access surgery is often replacing conventional surgery, but the equipment is often heat-labile and difficult to clean. All of these problems have been well addressed in this manual.

Litigation for negligence is becoming increasingly common and often involves possible deficiences in control of infection procedures. This further emphasises the importance of having well-defined procedures and ensuring that they are implemented by training of staff and audit.

The prevention of infection is one of the requirements for good quality of care of patients and is relevant to all members of staff. Protection of staff from infection is now a major consideration and is backed by health and safety legislation. Hospitals should have an infection control organisation which includes an infection control doctor, usually the medical microbiologist in the UK, and one or more infection control nurses, depending on the size of the hospital and the type of patient. These are members of the team who should meet daily or at least several times a week. The infection control committee is an expansion of the team and meets less frequently. It is important for approving policies and programmes, and for making recommendations which have a major financial implication to the Chief Executive. Collaboration with the community is also necessary and the Consultant in Communicable Disease Control (CCDC) should be a member of the infection control committee.

It is obviously necessary, in view of the problems described, for every hospital to have an infection control manual. To produce such a manual is a major task and it is time wasting for every hospital to produce it's own. This manual, originally produced by Dr Damani and his colleagues for Craigavon hospital, covers all the main policies required in a hospital. It has been expanded to include basic information on the various topics and is now generally applicable to other hospitals in the UK and many other countries. It will be particularly useful in countries or hospitals which are setting up new infection control programmes. However, although national and hospital guidelines are important, individual departments differ and the final decisions should be made by local infection control staff.

This manual contains a wealth of practical advice, a number of useful tables, diagrams, definitions and essential references. The policies are detailed and provide sufficient instructions to carry out individual procedures. Infection control staff will find this manual useful for producing shorter manuals for individual wards. These should be introduced as part of an ongoing educational programme to ensure the manuals are not only read but are followed by nursing and medical staff and administrators. The manual should also be useful in preparing audit programmes. I congratulate Dr Damani on producing a comprehensive and useful manual of procedures.

G. A. J. Ayliffe
1997

PREFACE

...by foreseeing in a distance, which is only done by men of talents, the evils which arise from them are soon cured; but when, from want of foresight, they are suffered to increase to such a height that they are perceptible to everyone, there is no remedy.

Niccolò Machiavelli

1513

Prevention of infection acquired in the health care setting remains a major goal for all health care personnel because of increased morbidity and mortality for patients. In addition, it utilizes resources that could be used elsewhere in health care.

Studies in the UK, Europe and North America indicate that approximately 10% of patients develop infection whilst in hospital. Evidence in the USA suggests that one third of hospital-acquired (nosocomial) infections could be prevented. Therefore financial benefit to the health care provider could be substantial by prevention of such infections.

Although in recent years there have been an increased allocation of resources directed to the problem of infection control services, the resources allocated have been constrained. This is because in the recent years the very nature of the hospital has changed. With the reduction in numbers of beds, the sickest patients have been concentrated in hospital and the throughput of patients has increased. Patients are often subjected to more aggressive diagnostic & therapeutic procedures and a greater number of health care workers are involved in the patient's management. In addition, newer varieties of the microorganisms are responsible for a wider spectrum of nosocomial infection, and bacterial isolates are becoming more resistant to the standard antibiotic therapies.

Although hospital-acquired infection has been worrying health care professionals for many years, more recently it is worrying patients and the public as well. This is due to emerging new pathogens coupled with heightened public awareness caused by AIDS, blood-borne hepatitis (B&C), methicillin resistant *Staph. aureus* (MRSA), and more recently by *Clostridium difficile*, multidrug resistant tuberculosis (MDR-TB), vancomycin resistant enterococci (VRE) and *E. coli* 0157 making their control more problematic and challenging for infection control personnel world wide.

Until the 1960s, recommendations on the control of infection were subjective, based on personal observations and anecdotes. The art beginning to emerge but the science was lacking. It is only in the past two decades that infection control has been taken as a serious issue although there are still areas where practice is still ritualist and controversial. An attempt has been made in this book to provide practical advice to the health care worker on the control of infection based on current scientific knowledge and recommendations from various bodies on prevention and control of infection in the health care setting.

Nizam N. Damani
1997

ACKNOWLEDGEMENTS

I wish to take this opportunity to thank the following people who have made the production of this book possible:

1. Jemima M. Keyes, Senior Nurse Infection Control, for Craigavon Area Hospital Group Trust who is also author of chapter 1 and is responsible for giving her precious time in reading the manuscript and making helpful comments and suggestions from her wide experience. I would also like to thank Dr. Peter Coyle, consultant virologist at the Royal Hospital Group, Belfast for his valuable comments on virology.

2. Linda McAlister, my secretary for her skill and energies for production of numerous drafts and maintenance of complicated correspondence and above all for her patience and missing numerous coffee breaks to meet the deadlines.

3. Derek Virtue of DataNet for design & production, Gavin Smith, Gavin Jamieson, and Geoffrey Nuttall of Greenwich Medical Media for seeing the book through completion.

4. Bayer AG, for giving permission to reproduce art work from *ARS Bacteriologica* based on the work of artist Carl W Röhring, for the title and back cover.

5. Finally, I thank my wife Laila and my children Numair and Namiz for their understanding and willingness to accommodate their life to my chaotic schedules.

CONTENTS

3 DISINFECTION POLICY

4 PREVENTION OF INFECTION CAUSED BY SPECIFIC PATHOGENS

ABBREVIATIONS

AAFB	Acid and Alcohol Fast Bacilli
ACDP	Advisory Committee on Dangerous Pathogens
AIDS	Acquired Immune Deficiency Syndrome
BS	British Standard
BBV	Blood-borne viruses
CCDC	Consultant in Communicable Disease Control
CDSC	Communicable Disease Surveillance Centre
CJD	Creutzfeldt-Jakob Disease
COSHH	Control of Substances Hazardous to Health
CSSD	Central Sterile Supplies Department
DHSS	Department of Health and Social Security
EHO	Environmental Health Officer
EL	Executive Letter
ELISA	Enzyme Linked Immunosorbent Assay
HAV	Hepatitis A Virus
HBIG	Hepatitis B Immunoglobulin

HBeAg	Hepatitis Be antigen
HBsAg	Hepatitis B surface antigen
HBV	Hepatitis B Virus
HC	Health Circular
HCV	Hepatitis C Virus
HIV	Human Immunodeficiency Virus
HMSO	Her Majesty's Stationery Office
HN	Health Notice
HSE	Health and Safety Executive
HSID	High Security Infectious Disease unit
HSG	Health Service Guidelines
ICC	Infection Control Committee
ICD	Infection Control Doctor
ICN	Infection Control Nurse
ICT	Infection Control Team
ICU	Intensive Care Unit
IV	Intravenous
MDA	Medical Device Agency
MRSA	Methicillin-resistant *Staphylococcus aureus*
NaDCC	Sodium Dichloroisocyanurate

OHD	Occupational Health Department	SCBU	Special Care Baby Unit
PCR	Polymerase Chain Reaction	VHF	Viral Haemorrhagic Fevers
PHLS	Public Health Laboratory Service	VRE	Vancomycin Resistant Enterococci
ppm av Cl$_2$	parts per million of available chlorine	VZIG	Varicella Zoster Immunoglobulin
QAC	Quatenary Ammonium Compound	VZV	Varicella Zoster Virus

GLOSSARY OF INFECTION CONTROL TERMS

ANTISEPSIS
The destruction or inhibition of micro-organisms on living tissues having the effect of limiting or preventing the harmful results of infection.

ANTISEPTIC
A chemical agent used in antisepsis.

CARRIER
A person (host) who harbours a micro-organism (agent) in the absence of discernible clinical disease. Carriers may shed organisms into environment intermittently or continuously and therefore act as a potential source of infection.

CASE
A person with symptoms.

CHEMOPROPHYLAXIS
The administration of antimicrobial agents to prevent the development of an infection or the progression of an infection to active manifest disease.

COHORT
A group of patients infected or colonized with same microorganism, grouped together in a designated area of a unit or ward.

COLONIZATION
The presence of microorganisms at a body site(s) without presence of symptoms or clinical manifestations of illness or infection. Colonization may be a form of carriage and is a potential method of transmission.

COMMENSAL
A microorganism resident in or on a body site without causing clinical infection.

COMMUNICABLE PERIOD

The time in the natural history of an infection during which transmission may take place.

CONTACT

An exposed individual who might have been infected through transmission from another host or the environment.

CONTAMINATION

The presence of microorganisms on a surface or in a fluid or material.

DISINFECTANT

A chemical agent which under defined conditions is capable of disinfection.

ENDEMIC

The usual level or presence of an agent or disease in a defined population during a given period.

ENDOGENOUS INFECTION

Microorganisms originating from the patient's own body which cause harm in another body site.

EPIDEMIC

An unusual, higher than expected level of infection or disease by a common agent in a defined population in a given period.

EPIDEMIOLOGY

The study of the occurrence and cause of disease in populations.

EXOGENOUS INFECTION

Microorganisms originating from a source or reservoir which are transmitted by any mechanism to a person, ie contact, airborne routes etc.

FLORA

Microorganisms resident in an environmental or body site.

HOSPITAL-ACQUIRED INFECTION
(nosocomial infection)

Infection acquired during hospitalization; not present or incubating at the time of admission to hospital.

IMMUNITY

The resistance of a host to a specific infectious agent.

IMMUNOCOMPROMISED

A state of reduced resistance to infection that results form malignant disease, drugs, radiation illness or congenital defect.

INCIDENCE The number of new cases of a disease (or event) occurring in a specified time.

INCIDENCE RATE The ratio of the number of new infections or disease in a defined population in a given period to the number of individuals at risk in the population.

INCUBATION PERIOD The time interval between initial exposure to the infectious agent and the appearance of the first sign or symptoms of the disease in a susceptible host.

INDEX CASE The first case to be recognized in a series of transmissions of an agent in a host population.

INFECTION The damaging of body tissue by microorganisms or by poisonous substances released by the microorganisms.

ISOLATION The physical separation of an infected or colonized host from the remainder of the at risk population in an attempt to prevent transmission of the specific agent to other individuals and patients.

MICROBIOLOGICAL CLEARANCE The reduction of the number of pathogenic microorganisms in a specimen below that detectable by conventional means.

MICROORGANISM A microscopic entity capable of replication. It includes bacteria, viruses and the microscopic forms of algae, fungi and protozoa.

OUTBREAK Two or more epidemiologically linked cases of infection caused by the same microorganism in place and/or time.

PATHOGEN A microorganism capable of producing disease.

PATHOGENICITY The ability of an infectious agent to cause disease in a susceptible host.

PREVALENCE RATE The ratio of the total number of individuals who have a disease at a particular time to the population at risk of having the disease.

RESERVOIR

Any animate or inanimate focus in the environment in which an infectious agent may survive and multiply and which may act as a potential source of infection.

SEROCONVERSION

The development of antibodies not previously present resulting from a primary infection.

SOURCE

Place where microorganisms are growing or have grown.

SPORADIC CASE

A single case which has not apparently been associated with other cases, excreters or carriers in the same period of time.

STERILE

Free from all living microorganisms.

STERILIZATION

A process which renders an item sterile.

STERILIZING AGENT
(Sterilant)

An agent or combination of agents which under defined conditions leads to sterilization.

SURVEILLANCE

A systematic collection, analysis and interpretation of data on specific events (infections) and disease, followed by dissemination of that information to those who can improve the outcomes.

SUSCEPTIBLE

A person presumably not possessing sufficient resistance (or immunity) against a pathogenic agent who contracts infection when exposed to the agent.

TRANSMISSION

The method by which any potentially infecting agent is spread to another host.

VIRULENCE

The intrinsic capabilities of a microorganism to infect host and produce disease.

ZOONOSIS

An infectious disease transmissible from vertebrate animals to humans.

1

ORGANISATION OF INFECTION CONTROL PROGRAMME

In the UK the organisation of an infection control programme is based on the joint recommendations of the Department of Health and Public Health Laboratories Services guidelines on the Hospital Infection Control (The Cooke Report). In summary, it recommends that each major hospital should have an Infection Control Team and an Infection Control Committee. The Infection Control Committee advises the chief executive on the control of hospital infection and together they agree on resources needed for the day to day running of the infection control programme and contingency plan for an outbreak. Guidance is also given as to the recommended structure, roles and responsibilities of those persons directly involved in the planning and implementation of an effective infection control programme. The report also highlights that the chief executive of the each hospital has an overall responsibility for the provision of infection control in their Trust. He or she also has an overall responsibility for ensuring that this is facilitated primarily by allocation of adequate resources and managerially ensuring that full support is afforded to the infection control team to implement the infection control programme effectively.

It is important to emphasize that in order to establish an effective infection control programme it not only requires adequate funding, but also the employment of personnel with specialist knowledge, practical experience and adequate training.

INFECTION CONTROL DOCTOR

The Infection Control Doctor must be a registered medical practitioner and should have an experience in the medical microbiology and epidemiology of hospital infection and in the methods for its prevention and control. He or she is most likely to be a consultant medical microbiologist, but hospital consultants in other disciplines (eg infectious diseases) may be appointed. The Infection Control Doctor is managerially accountable to the chief executive of the hospital, and professionally to the Medical Director or as otherwise decided by the employer. The role and responsibility of the Infection Control Doctor is summarised as follows:

- Serves as a specialist advisor and takes a leading role in the effective functioning of the Infection Control Team.

- Should be an active member of the hospital Infection Control Committee and may act as its Chairman.

- Assists the hospital Infection Control Committee in drawing up annual plans, policies and long-term programmes for the prevention of hospital infection.

- Advises the chief executive directly on all aspects of infection control in the hospital and on the implementation of agreed policies.

- Participates in the preparation of the tender documents for support services and advises on infection control aspects.

- Involved in setting quality standards with regard to hospital infection and in the audit of infection.

- Serves as an active member on the District/Area Infection Control Committee.

INFECTION CONTROL NURSE

An Infection Control Nurse is a registered nurse with an additional academic education and practical training which enables him or her to act as a specialist advisor in all matters relating to infection control. A recognised qualification in infection control should be held which will allow recognition of the Infection Control Nurse as a specialist practitioner.

The Infection Control Nurse is usually the only full-time practitioner in the Infection Control Team and therefore takes the key role in day to day infection control activities, with the Infection Control Doctor providing the lead role. The role and responsibility of the Infection Control Nurse is summarised as follows :

- Serves as a specialist advisor and takes a leading role in the effective functioning of the Infection Control Team.

- Should be an active member of the hospital Infection Control Committee.

- Assists the hospital Infection Control Committee in drawing up annual plans and policies for infection control.

- Provide specialist nursing input in the identification, prevention, monitoring and control of infection within the hospital.

- Surveillance, investigation and the control of infection in the hospital.

- Identify, investigate and monitor infections, hazardous practice and procedures.

- Advise the contracting departments, participating in the preparation of documents relating to service specifications and quality standards.

- Ongoing contribution in development and implementation of infection control policy & procedure, participating in audit, and monitoring tools related to infection control and infectious diseases.

- Presentation of educational programmes and membership of relevant committees where infection control input is required.

It is essential that the Infection Control Nurse should have an expert knowledge of both general and specialist nursing practice and must also have an understanding not only of the functioning of clinical areas but also operational areas and services. He or she must also be able to communicate effectively with all grades of staff, negotiate and effect change, and influence practice.

CONSULTANT IN COMMUNICABLE DISEASE CONTROL

The Consultant in Communicable Disease Control (CCDC) is appointed by the Department of Public Health Medicine for the surveillance, prevention and control of communicable diseases and infection within the boundaries of a Regional Health Authority or Area Board. In most places the CCDC is proper officer under the Public Health (Control of Diseases) Act 1984 by formal appointment of the Local Authority. CCDC acts on behalf of the Director of Public Health which enables him or her to make executive decisions in all matters relevant to communicable disease control in the interest of protecting the health of the general population.

Whilst the CCDC is generally held to be responsible for ensuring that adequate arrangements for the prevention of communicable disease and infection control in the community are made, the Infection Control Team have this responsibility within the acute sector. The CCDC liaises with the hospital Infection Control Team, receiving such information on matters of infection and transmissible disease which are relative to the community as a whole. The interest and the role of the CCDC in hospital infection control is summarised as follows:

- Advise purchasers on appropriate contractual requirement relating to infection control services and on monitoring the contracts and any other relevant arrangements.

- Liaise with Infection Control Team to make a judgement on the implications of hospital infections/outbreaks for the community, on the implications of community based outbreaks for the hospital, and to take appropriate action.

- To provide epidemiological advice whenever it is needed, both routinely and in outbreaks.

- Through chairmanship of the District/Area Infection Control Committee to facilitate liaison with other Infection Control Teams in the area and with other local agencies, and to develop common policies and procedures.

The CCDC is the link between the Health Service and the local Health Authority/Area Health Board in the control of communicable disease. It is important that he or she should be aware of problems within the hospital that may have implications for the local community. Close collaboration between the CCDC and the Infection Control Team on a regular basis is essential if both are to contribute fully to efforts to prevent communicable disease and infection inside and outside hospitals.

INFECTION CONTROL TEAM

The Infection Control Team comprises of the Infection Control Doctor and Infection Control Nurse. The Infection Control Doctor is usually a consultant medical microbiologist; if this is not the case, this person should be added to the team. The Infection Control Team is responsible for the day to day running of infection control programmes.

All acute hospitals should have an Infection Control Team, although smaller health care providers may not find this a viable option. In cases where the provision of an Infection Control Team is not practical, arrangements for the provision of and access to the infection control service should formally be made with a local acute hospital.

The role of the Infection Control Team is to ensure that an effective infection control programme has been planned, co-ordinate its implementation, and evaluate the impact of such measures. Whilst they will actively participate in most of these areas, some aspects of the infection control programme may fall under the remit of others. In such cases the Infection Control Team will provide advice and direction, ultimately ensuring that all tasks reach completion. It is important to ensure that there is provision made for 24 hour access to the Infection Control Team for advice on infection prevention and control of infection which would include both medical and nursing advice. The role of the Infection Control Team can be summarized as follows :

- Production of an annual infection control programme with clearly defined objectives.

- Production of written policies and procedures on infection control, including regular evaluation and update.

- Education of all grades of staff in infection control policy, practice and procedures relevant to their own area of practice.

- Surveillance of infection to detect outbreaks at the earliest opportunity and provide data which should be evaluated to allow for any change in practice or allocation of resource to prevent hospital acquired infections.

- Provide advice to all grades of staff on all matters in relation to infection prevention and control on a day to day basis.

INFECTION CONTROL COMMITTEE

The hospital Infection Control Committee is charged with the responsibility for the planning, evaluation and implementation of all matters relating to infection control, the making of major decisions and resource allocation playing a major part in this.

The membership of the hospital Infection Control Committee may vary according to local arrangements for infection control provision. The following membership is recommended:

- Infection Control Doctor (chairperson).

- Infection Control Nurse.

- Chief executive or his or her nominated representative.

- Consultant in Communicable Disease Control.

- The clinical directors of the hospital representing major clinical specialties, including an Infectious Diseases Physician, if one is available.

- The Director of Nursing or a representative.

- An Occupational Health Physician or a representative.

Additionally, representatives of any other department may be invited as necessary. The Infection Control Committee should meet regularly according to local need. A minimum of two planned meetings a year is recommended. The Committee may, at the request of the Chairperson, be convened at any other time to deal with serious infection control problems and in an outbreak situation.

The function of the local Infection Control Committee is that of supporting the development of an effective infection control programme. It is important that the members of the committee voice areas of concern and any problems relating to either infection control practice or policy, in particular highlighting areas which have not been addressed within their own sphere of responsibility. The committee should discuss implications, approve infection control policies and assist in their implementation.

SURVEILLANCE

A surveillance programme, which includes the collection of data on infections, analysis to determine the significance and identify any factors which may prevent infection, is necessary for an effective infection control programme. The most vital component, however, is ensuring that the information obtained is conveyed to those who may influence practice, implement change or provide financial resources necessary to improve outcomes. In summary, it is a futile exercise to collect and record data without taking any further action. Surveillance data is a useful tool for both the Infection Control Team and the Infection Control Committee to identify areas of priority and allocate resources accordingly. Therefore, the main objectives of surveillance are:

- To identify cases or potential cases of transmissible infections.

- To facilitate the relevant investigations and implement infection control measures to minimize their incidence.

- To detect and predict trends and seasonal variations and make arrangements to implement the relevant infection control measures.

- To ascertain trends in the actual occurrence of transmissible infections on an annual basis, to facilitate the allocation of resources to implement the relevant infection control measures.

- To identify infection control problems which may be remedied in order to prevent a recurrence.

The process of surveillance must incorporate four key stages: data must be **collected**, **recorded**, **analyzed**, **interpreted** in the light of local circumstances, and finally presented to those who are in a position to take the necessary action.

Many different methods of surveillance exist; a recent study examined some of these methods and the finding are summarised in table 1.1. Local factors,

Table 1.1– Various methods of surveillance used in infection control.

Method	Sources of data	Comments
Continuing surveillance of all patients (CS).	Medical, nursing, laboratory records including temperature charts, X-ray and antibiotics treatment reports.	Time-consuming and not cost-effective: infection rates are low in some specialties.
Ward liaison (WL).	Twice-weekly visits to wards. Discuss all patients with staff and review records.	Less comprehensive than CS, with similar disadvantages.
Laboratory-based (LB).	Laboratory records only.	Depends on samples taken and information on request forms.
Laboratory-based ward surveillance (LBWS).	Follow up of LB in wards.	Disadvantages of LB, but more accurate.
Laboratory-based ward surveillance and selected continuing surveillance (LBWS+CS).	As LBWS and reporting of outbreaks by ward staff and CS in special units (eg ITU) or infections (eg wounds).	As LBWS, but early detection of outbreaks and incidence studies in selected areas of infection.
Laboratory-based ward liason (LBWL).	Combination of LB and LBWS.	Time-consuming but most sensitive after CS.

Adapted and reproduced with permission from Glenister HM *et al*. An evaluation of surveillance methods for detecting infections in hospital inpatients. *J Hosp Infect* 1993; **23**: 229-242. and from Ayliffe GAJ, Babb JR. *Pocket Reference to Hospital-acquired Infection*. London: Science Press, 1995:13.

including the priorities set by the Infection Control Committee and the allocation of resources to the Infection Control Team will influence the surveillance method chosen. Surveillance and data collection by the Infection Control Team is necessary to detect and monitor outbreaks.

The efficacy of an infection control surveillance programme will ultimately depend on the resources allocated. Such factors as personnel, training, resources within the Infection Control Department, including adequate access to computer systems, playing a major part. The final decision as to which method of surveillance process should be adopted rests with the Infection Control Team and the Infection Control Committee.

MANAGEMENT OF MAJOR OUTBREAK

In 1986 the report of the committee of inquiry into an outbreak of food poisoning at the Stanley Royd Hospital recommended that each district should prepare a plan for dealing with a major outbreak of food poisoning or communicable disease. Subsequent reports of outbreaks of infectious disease, including Legionnaire's, have highlighted the need for appropriate planning to effectively manage such episodes. Among the most frequent issues of concern addressed in these reports have been those of individual responsibilities, relationships and communications. Given these concerns, there is a need for formulating outbreak control plans by each Health Authority or Area Board.

The concept of a major outbreak is unsatisfactory as often this can only be a retrospective assessment. To try to identify a major outbreak in terms of number of cases fails to recognise the elementary fact that, from the point of view of infectious disease control, a single case of viral haemorrhagic fever or few cases of Legionnaires' still warrants full major outbreak planning. Therefore, a major incident or outbreak is not dependant so much on the numbers of people affected but rather the nature of the infectious agent, the pathogenicity and the transmissibility of the microorganism. The occurrence of a major incident or outbreak should therefore be determined locally by the Infection Control Doctor (ICD) and/or the Consultant in Communicable Disease Control (CCDC). Day to day surveillance is important to identify infectious diseases so that appropriate action is taken. Major outbreaks of transmissible infection in both the hospital and community require appropriate planning to ensure effective management of such episodes. There must be a written policy which clearly addresses the areas of individual responsibilities, and action plans for all involved. Those who are or may be involved in the management of a major outbreak must be aware of such a policy and their individual role.

It is the responsibility of the Infection Control Committee, in liaison with the CCDC, to draw up detailed plans appropriate to local situations, and particular units for the management of the incidents and outbreak in the hospital. These plans should be discussed and endorsed by the hospital Infection Control Committee and should include the criteria and method for convening the Outbreak Control Group which, when necessary, will be expanded into a Major Outbreak Control (Group) Committee. There should be one clearly identified person taking the leading role in the management of any outbreak. Although the ICD will take the lead in most incidents or outbreaks in hospital, there will be those in which it will still be more appropriate for the CCDC to take the initiative. If the outbreak begins in the community and then affects the hospital, the CCDC will already be in control.

Notification

Medical staff have a statutory duty to give notification of certain infectious diseases which are diagnosed or suspected in patients whom they are attending, to the CCDC. Telephone reporting of infections with serious implications for Public Health, whether or not they are legally notifiable is important. It is the responsibility of both medical and nursing staff that if they suspect an incident of communicable disease or food poisoning in a ward, hospital or health care facility, they report this immediately to the ICD and/or CCDC.

Recognition

The rapid recognition of outbreaks is one of the most important objectives of the routine surveillance of infection. Sometimes the outbreak may manifest itself clearly to the medical and nursing staff, who must inform the Infection Control Team of its occurrence. However, some outbreaks may arise more insidiously and reach considerable proportions before they become apparent. These outbreaks are detected by the laboratory, but under some circumstances may be identified only through the vigilance of general nursing and medical staff both in hospital and the community. These must notified to the Infection Control Team and the CCDC. The local authority Environmental Health Officer should be informed promptly of any infectious incident where food or water is implicated.

Investigation

Once a possible outbreak has been recognised, the ICD is the person primarily responsible for action within the hospital. The ICD and ICN will take immediate steps to collect information from the ward and the laboratory, determine whether an outbreak is occurring and establish a case definition. If the initial investigation confirms that an outbreak is occurring it is important to establish its severity and initiate some immediate control measures. If after the initial observation it is established that no outbreak exists then it is important that the person who has made the initial observation should be informed and the reason given. Ward staff may need reassurance and care should be taken not to discourage further reporting. In the community the CCDC will make the necessary preliminary investigations and consultations to determine whether or not there is an outbreak and decide on appropriate action.

Table 1.2 – Summary for investigation of an outbreak.

- Confirm the existence of an outbreak.
- Verify the diagnosis.
- Create a case definition.
- Identify and count cases or exposures.
- Develop a hypothesis (eg mode of spead, reservoir).
- Develop a line-listing.
- Tabulate and set the data in terms of time, place and person.
- Take immediate control measures.
- Communicate information to relevant personnel.
- Screening of personnel and evironment as indicated.
- Write a coherent report (preliminary and final).
- Summarize investigation and recommendations to the appropriate authorities.

Outbreak Control Plan

The decision to convene an Outbreak Control Group should be made by ICD and CCDC, depending upon the nature of the infectious disease and number of cases involved. The Outbreak Control Group generally consists of ICD, ICN, chief executive or representative, CCDC, senior nurse and clinician in charge.

The aim of the Outbreak Control Group is to:

- Facilitate the investigation of the outbreak.
- Implement measures necessary to control the outbreak.
- Monitor the effectiveness of the control measures.
- Oversee communication to all relevant groups.
- Facilitate the medical care of patients.

Each member of the Outbreak Control Group should have an "Action Card" to outline his or her responsibilities and duties, and to act as a check list of tasks to be considered. The Chairman of the group should have a complete set of cards so as to be aware of the responsibilities of each member of the Group. If there is a major incident, such as a substantial outbreak of food poisoning or a case of an unusual communicable disease, the Outbreak Control Group should expand to form a Major Outbreak Control (Group) Committee and seek advice from experts both at local and national levels. Advice is available from the Public Health Laboratory Service, Communicable Disease Surveillance Centre (CDSC), telephone 0171-200-6868 or the Scottish Centre for Infection and Environmental Health, telephone 0141-946-7120. They provide advice on a 24-hour basis and can provide personnel if invited.

Communication

The Outbreak Control Group will inform the senior management of the hospital and other appropriate people on a regular basis. They should also liaise with the CDSC, Public Health Laboratory Service, General Practitioners, Department of Health, other Directors of Public Health and the Chief Medical Officer.

In an outbreak situation, it is good practice to have one designated person within the health care facility to respond to the inquiries from the public, press and the media. That person should be kept informed of all the developments by the chair-person of the Outbreak Control Group.

End of outbreak

At the end of an outbreak the Outbreak Control Group will prepare a final report. When the outbreak has been controlled, a final meeting of the Outbreak Control Group should be held to:

- Review the experience of all participants involved in management of outbreak.

- Identify any shortfalls and particular difficulties that were encountered.

- Revise the outbreak control plan in accordance with the results.

- Recommend, if necessary, structural or procedural improvements which would reduce the chances of recurrence.

References and further reading

Department of Health and Public Health Laboratory Services. *Hospital Infection Control: Guidance on the control of infection in hospitals* (The Cooke Report). London: Department of Health, 1995.

Department of Health and Public Health Medicine Environmental Group. *Guidelines on the Control of Infection in Residential and Nursing Homes*. London: Department of Health, 1996.

Department of Health and Social Security. Public Health in England. *The Report of an Enquiry into the Future Development of the Public Health Function*. (The Acheson Report). London: HMSO, 1988.

Association of Medical Microbiologists, Hospital Infection Society, Infection Control Nurses Association and Public Health Laboratory Services. The Infection Control Standards Working Party. *Standards in Infection Control in Hospitals*. London: HMSO, 1993.

Glenister HM, Taylor LJ, Cooke EM, Bartlett CLR. *A Study of Surveillance Methods for Detecting Hospital Infection*. London: Public Health Laboratory Services, 1992.

Emmerson AM, Ayliffe GAJ. Surveillance of Nosocomial Infections. *Clinical Infectious Diseases* 1996; **3(2)**: 159-301.

Haley RW, Culver DH, White JW. The efficacy of infection surveillance and control programs in preventing nosocomial infection in US hospitals. (SENIC study). *American Journal of Epidemiology* 1985; **121(2)**: 182-205.

Glynn A, Ward V, Wilson J *et al*. *Hospital-Aquired Infection: Surveillance, Policies and Practice*. London: Public Health Laboratory Services, 1997.

Emmerson AM, Enstone JE, Griffin M *et al*. The Second National Prevalence Survey of Infection in Hospitals – overview of the results. *Journal of Hospital Infection* 1996; **32:** 175-190.

2

ISOLATION POLICY
FOR PATIENTS WITH
INFECTIOUS DISEASES

Routes of transmission of infection have been understood for many years and this knowledge has been used to develop policies and procedures on isolation of patients with communicable disease or epidemiologically important microorganisms. All health care workers who are in direct contact with the patients in isolation have a responsibility to observe the precautions outlined in the policy. It is important to emphasise that isolation precautions can protect only if they are used consistently and appropriately. Hospitals are directed to develop a system to ensure that patients, personnel, and visitors are educated about the use of precautions and their responsibility to adhere to them. Hospitals are also directed to evaluate adherence to precautions and to use findings to direct improvements.

Infection control measures outlined in this chapter are designed to intercept the route of transmission of infection, therefore the correct application of infection control procedures requires a knowledge of the infecting microorganism, mode of transmission and susceptibility of the host. The policy for patients in isolation is based on a two tier precautions system. The first tier precautions contain routine infection control precautions (see page 15) that are designed for the care of all patients regardless of their diagnosis or presumed infectious status. The second tier of precaution is based on the transmission of infection and is designed to supplement the routine infection control precautions which should be used for patients known or suspected to be infected/colonized with the transmissible or epidemiologically important microorganisms. The second tier precautions are grouped into various categories according to mode of transmission. It is important to emphasise that some microorganisms have more that one mode of transmission and, therefore, more than one category of source isolation precautions may be used. In such cases advice from a member of the local Infection Control Team should be sought and isolation precautions should be modified according to local needs. The following points are common to all categories of isolation precautions:

1. All patients with suspected/proven infection should be isolated in a side ward. If a separate room is not available, seek advice from a member of the Infection Control Team regarding patient placement. In some cases the patient may be nursed in an open ward provided that the isolation is followed meticulously. but this is the least favourable option. The patient can be accommodated at one end of the ward, close to the washhand basin and sluice. If more than one patient is affected (eg in an outbreak), they should be cohorted in a single cubicle/area and looked after by dedicated nursing staff.

2. All visitors must report to the nurse-in-charge before entering the room about instruction on protective clothing and other precautions.

3. Wash hands immediately to avoid transfer of microorganisms to other patients or environment.

4. If possible, attend the patient in source isolation last, after dealing with all non-infected patients.

5. If common equipment is unavoidable, items must be adequately cleaned and disinfected, preferably by heat, before use on other patients.

6. Room should be terminally cleaned (see page 71) after discharge of the patient with infective condition or epidemiologically important microorganism.

7. It is important to consider the psychological effect of isolation on patients and a member of the Infection Control Team should discuss concerns expressed by the patient or their family members.

PROTECTIVE CLOTHING

Personal protective clothing is used in the health care setting to prevent cross-infection between patients and health care workers. Protective clothing which conforms to British Standards or other international standards should be used, where possible.

Gloves: Single-use disposable sterile gloves should be used during aseptic procedures to prevent patients acquiring infection from the health care worker. Non-sterile gloves should be used for all procedures involving contact with blood, body fluids, excretions and secretions where there is a risk of infection to the health care worker and asepsis is not necessary.

Non-disposable household or heavyweight type gloves are required for environmental cleaning and decontamination procedures because they are robust and offer greater protection to the health care worker in these procedures. They should be washed and dried after each use and must be discarded if punctured or heavily contaminated with infected material. Heavy duty gloves are required for those situations where additional protection is required eg handling clinical waste bags prior to final disposal to minimize risk of injury to the health care worker.

Aprons and gowns: Single-use disposable plastic aprons or gowns should be worn during procedures that are likely to generate splashes of blood or body fluids or activities that may contaminate clothes or uniforms from microorganisms or infectious material. They are available in two lengths ie short length (above the knee) and long length (to the ankle). They should be removed immediately after use by tearing the neck strap and the waist tie and discarded into a clinical waste bag before they leave the room.

Face protection: Use masks alone when there is a risk of respiratory transmission of infectious agent. Masks in conjunction with eyewear should be worn during procedures that are likely to generate aerosols or splashes of blood and body fluids to prevent contamination of mucous membranes of the mouth, nose and eyes. Thin surgical masks provide minimal protection against air borne pathogens. However if they are recommended for use, then for maximum efficiency, they should be close fitting with filter particles size of <5 microns should be used.

If the masks are used then they should be used only once and changed when moist or grossly contaminated. Masks should be removed by untying and handled only by the ties and never by the face covering part which may be heavily contaminated with the microorganisms.

Overshoes: The use of overshoes is not recommended as it is an ideal way of transferring microorganisms from floor and shoes to hands.

SUMMARY OF ROUTINE INFECTION CONTROL PRECAUTIONS

Isolation of patients

All patients with known or suspected infection should be isolated in a single side room with en suite toilet facilities. This should be done at the time of admission. Appropriate infection precautions must commence on clinical suspicion; laboratory confirmation is not necessary. If the single room is not available then patients with same infection or colonized with the same microorganisms may be cohorted in a designated area; this is particularly useful in an outbreak situation. Cohorting of patients should always be done on the advice of a member of the local Infection Control Team. Limited movement and transport of these patients is essential ensuring that they leave their room only for essential, purposes to minimize spread in the hospital. If transport of such patients is necessary, seek advice from a member of the Infection Control Team.

Notification

Medical practitioners attending patients with known or suspected to be suffering from a communicable disease have a statutory obligation to inform the Consultant in Communicable Disease Control both in the hospital and community. In hospital, it is important that all such cases are also notified to a member of the Infection Control Team. This should be done as soon as possible, preferably by phone if the suspected disease concerned is of a serious nature, to ensure a speedy and proper follow-up and, in cases of suspected outbreak, prompt investigation to prevent further spread. Notification should occur on clinical suspicion of the disease and is **not** dependent on laboratory confirmation.

Hand washing

Hand washing is the single most important method to prevent cross infection. They should be washed regularly between patients and procedures and after contact with blood, body fluids, excretion, secretion and after contact with contaminated items. Hands should be washed immediately after gloves are removed.

Cover cuts

Cover cuts or areas of broken skin with waterproof dressings whilst at work. Health care workers with large areas of broken skin must avoid invasive procedures. Staff with eczema or other skin conditions or with large wounds which cannot be adequately protected by plastic gloves or impermeable dressings should refrain from patient care and handling patient care equipment until the condition resolves. All staff with skin lesions should be referred to the Occupational Health Department for advice.

Wear protective clothing

Appropriate protective gear, ie masks, gowns, protective eye wear etc, should be worn for the procedures that are likely to generate droplets, splashes, or sprays of blood or body fluids to protect mucous membrane and skin.

Safe use of sharps

Avoid sharps usage wherever possible; if necessary they must be used and handled with care. Used needles must not be resheathed unless there is a safe means available for doing so. Do not bend, break or manipulate used needles by hand. A one-handed scoop technique or a mechanical device for holding of/disposing of needles may be used. Never leave sharps lying around; dispose of them carefully into a designated sharps container. Remember that it is the **personal responsibility** of the person using a sharp to dispose of it safely as soon as possible after use or ensure that it has been safely discarded. The sharps container must be closed securely when three-quarters full and disposed of by incineration. They must be labelled with the name of the health care facility, hospital and ward. They must be kept in a location which excludes injury to patients, visitors and staff.

Sharp injury

Sharps injury and accidental exposure of non-intact skin, conjunctiva or mucous membrane to blood or high risk body fluids must be recorded and reported to the Local Occupational Health Department or the Accident & Emergency Department according to the local policy.

Staff health

It is important that staff are appropriately and adequately immunized against infectious diseases, both for their own protection and the protection of others. Staff suffering from a known or suspected infectious disease must report this to the local Occupational Health Department who will advise on the management and exclusion from work, if required. Personal medical details will remain confidential to the Occupational Health Department.

Spillage of blood and body fluids

Spillage of blood and body fluids must be disinfected and cleaned promptly using a safe method (see page 70). Appropriative protective clothing must be worn and waste must be discarded as clinical waste.

Cleaning and disinfection of equipment

Patient care equipment is either single-use disposable or re-usable. Single-use items should be discarded as clinical waste while non-disposable equipment which is re-used between patients should be appropriately cleaned and disinfected or sterilized before re-use, according to the local policy.

Clinical waste

Waste from patients with a known or suspected infection should be treated as clinical waste and must be put into a yellow plastic bag. This must be securely fastened when three-quarters full, taken to a designated storage area for clinical waste from which they should be collected for incineration. Identification tag with name of the health care facility/hospital and ward should be marked on the clinical waste bag.

Laundry

Linen must be processed in accordance with the policy. Soiled linen should be handled with a minimum of agitation and placed in a laundry bag. Linen from infected patients should be placed in a water soluble stitched bag which is then placed in a second red bag and sealed at the door of the room. The bag should be labelled as infected linen "Danger of Infection". The name of the ward and date must also be written on the bag. All linen should be transported in a safe manner.

Environmental cleaning

Special attention must be given to the environment which should be maintained in a clean state, in line with good housekeeping practice. Terminal cleaning of the room should be carried out at the discharge of the patient using appropriate detergent/disinfectant solution (see page 71). Once the room is clean and dry, it can be used for other patients. Where special cleaning arrangements are required, the domestic services supervisor must be informed of the infection risk (not the patient's diagnosis) and any protective measures necessary for the staff.

Laboratory specimens

It is important that specimens should be taken before starting antibiotic therapy. Laboratory specimens must be correctly labelled and packaged, ie the request form must be kept separate from the specimen in a self-sealing plastic bag.

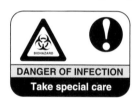

Specimens must be handled carefully ensuring that the outside of the container is not contaminated. Specimens from a patient with known or suspected infectious disease must have a "Danger of Infection – Take special care" label both on the request form and on the specimen.

All specimens must be transported in an appropriate container to the laboratory. The specimens from a patient known, or suspected, to be infected with highly transmissible and dangerous pathogens must not be sent to the laboratory without prior arrangement with the consultant microbiologist/clinical pathologist and/or the laboratory staff.

Written policy

Each health care facility should have a written policy and procedure manual on matters relating to control of infection to comply with Health & Safety Work Act, COSHH and other regulations.

Education and training

All staff, including those new to the post, must receive education and training in safe handling and disposal of sharps, infected waste and all other activities to prevent exposure of microorganisms to themselves and others. In addition, relevant staff should also be trained in aseptic techniques. The education programme should be regularly updated in view of changing knowledge and work practice. Written records should be kept by the ward manager.

Deceased patients

As a general rule the infection control precautions prescribed during life are continued after death. In cases where there is an infection risk from the body, a "Danger of Infection" label must be attached to the patient's arm band.

If a person known or suspected to be infected dies either in hospital or elsewhere, it is the duty of those with knowledge of the case to ensure that those who handle the body should be aware that there is a potential risk of infection, so that they may be protected by using the appropriate control measures. Making a known or suspected hazard known to those concerned is a statutory duty under the Health and Safety at Work Act.

HEALTH AND SAFTEY AT WORK ACT

All employers (including independent contractors) have a legal obligation under the Health and Safety at Work Act (1974) to ensure that all their employees are appropriately trained and proficient in the procedures necessary for working safely. They also have a responsibility to protect voluntary workers. Health and Safety at Work legislation also places a responsibility on employees to take all reasonable steps while at work to ensure their own health and safety, and those who may be affected by their acts or omissions at work. In addition, employers are required by the Control of Substances Hazardous to Health, (COSHH) Regulations (1988) to review every procedure carried out by the employee which involves contact with a substance hazardous to health, including pathogenic microorganisms.

CATEGORIES OF ISOLATION

Isolation procedures can be divided into two main categories:

Source isolation

The aim is to prevent the transfer of microorganisms from infected patients, who may act as a source of infection to staff or other patients. A side ward with its own toilet facilities is suitable for most type of patients in source isolation but for certain types of infectious diseases the room should be at negative pressure ventilation. Table 2.1 (see page 33) lists alphabetically the infection which require one of the isolation procedures with brief comments for further information.

Protective isolation

It should be used for severely immunocompromised patients who are highly susceptible to and need protection from infection from, both persons and the environment. A side room for protective isolation should preferably be at a positive pressure ventilation.

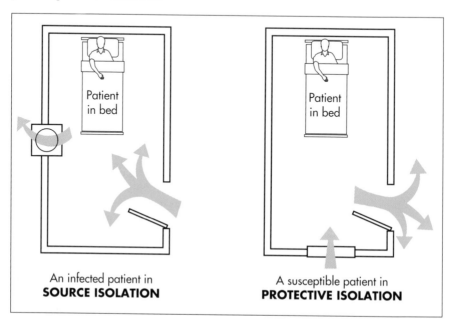

An infected patient in
SOURCE ISOLATION

A susceptible patient in
PROTECTIVE ISOLATION

STRICT ISOLATION

This is used to prevent transmission of diseases spread both by air and contact and used for patients with highly transmissible and dangerous infections, eg Lassa and other viral haemorrhagic fevers, pneumonic plague, pharyngeal diphtheria, etc. Patients requiring strict isolation must be admitted or transferred to a regional Infectious Diseases Unit in an ambulance with special precautions. Arrangements for such transfers must be made under the direct supervision of the Infection Control Doctor or Consultant in Communicable Disease Control.

Location   Patients must be admitted into a single room under negative pressure ventilation, with an ante room with wash hand basin and *en suite* toilet facilities.

The door must be kept closed except during necessary entrances and exits.

Remove any unnecessary items of equipment before the patient occupies the room.

Check that the mattress and pillows have non-permeable intact covers.

Ensure that disposable paper towels are available and an antiseptic/detergent hand cleanser is provided in an elbow operated pump dispenser.

Use disposable crockery and cutlery where possible.

Supply a large foot operated disposal bin lined with a yellow plastic bag for clinical waste.

Patient's charts should be kept outside the room.

Staff

Restrict the number of staff having access to the patient and the ward manager must maintain a list of all staff who have contact with the patient in strict isolation.

Visitors

They must be kept to a minimum and must always report to the sister or nurse-in-charge before entering the room and must observe the same infection control precautions as the staff.

Protective Clothing

Gloves: Well fitting, non-sterile single-use, disposable gloves must be worn, before entering the room, for direct patient care activity or when the contamination of hands are likely from the environment. The glove must cover the cuffs of the non-permeable long sleeved gown. They should be carefully removed and then discarded into the waste bin as clinical waste.

Gowns: Only disposable gowns with non-permeable fronts and sleeves must be used. Remove after use and discard into a clinical waste bag before leaving the room.

Masks: Only a high filtration mask which covers the nose and mouth should be worn. It must be put on before entering the room and removed before leaving and discarded into a clinical waste bag. The mask should be removed by untying the ties at the back and be handled and discarded by the ties only.

Eye Protection: Eye protection must be worn for any procedure which may cause splashes of blood and body fluids.

Other Protective Clothing: Protective footwear such as water-proof boots may be worn in situations where excessive exposure to blood and body fluids is anticipated.

Hand hygiene

Careful hand washing before leaving the room is most important. Hands must be washed with an antiseptic/ detergent preparation and dried thoroughly with a disposable paper towel. They must be washed after touching the patient or potentially contaminated articles and after removing protective clothing, eg gloves, gowns, masks etc.

When leaving the room the door should be pushed open from the outside by an assistant in order to avoid touching the door handle which may be contaminated. When outside, repeat the hand disinfection with alcoholic-chlorhexidine disinfection "Hibisol" to cleanse skin.

Equipment

Use disposable equipment wherever possible.

Any equipment or items required for patient care which are not disposable must be kept inside the patient's room.

No equipment or items should be returned for communal use without consulting a member of the Infection Control Team.

Laundry

Use disposable bed linen, if available. Non-disposable linen must be treated as infected linen and sterilized before processing in the laundry. Inform the CSSD and the laundry manager. In situations where this facility does not exist, the linen must be destroyed by incineration.

Decontamination & waste disposal

Used CSSD Equipment: Should be placed in an appropriate container and sealed. The CSSD manager must be contacted before further processing.

Domestic Cleaning: Seek advice from a member of the Infection Control Team.

Waste: All waste must be disposed of as clinical waste according to the local policy.

Body fluid spills

Spills of blood and body fluids must be immediately disinfected and cleaned (see page 70).

Inter-departmental visits

The patient must not leave the room without prior consultation with the Infection Control Doctor.

Laboratory specimens

They must not be taken or sent to the laboratory without prior discussion with the consultant microbiologist/ clinical pathologist, the CCDC or consultant physician in infectious disease.

The laboratory should be warned that they are about to receive a specimen from a patient with a highly dangerous infection.

Laboratory specimens must be correctly labelled and packaged, ie the request form must be kept separate from the specimen in a plastic bag. Specimens from patients with known or suspected infectious diseases must have a "Danger of Infection - Take special care" label both on the request form and on the specimen. All specimens must be transported to the laboratory in an appropriate container.

Last offices

The infection control measures employed during life must be continued after death. Only minimal handling of the body by trained personnel is permissible. Any bleeding part must be covered with an occlusive dressing. Appropriate personnel must be informed about the infectious status of the body.

The body must be transported in an appropriate sealed cadaver bag and must be labelled conspicuously with a "Danger of Infection" sticker on the identity band, the wrapping sheet or shroud and on the outside of the cadaver bag. The body *must not* be embalmed.

RESPIRATORY ISOLATION

This is used for infections which are transmitted by droplet nuclei. Droplets are generated in the course of talking, coughing, or sneezing and during procedures involving the respiratory tract such as suction, physiotherapy, intubation, or bronchoscopy. The size of droplets generated by these activity can either be small or large.

Small droplet nuclei size of $\leq 5\mu$ or smaller in size. These can be widely dispersed by air currents and reach alveoli of the recipient to cause infection. Diseases in this category include tuberculosis, varicella (chickenpox or disseminate varicella infection) and measles. The patient should be in a single room with negative airflow ventilation in relation to the surrounding areas. The door should be kept closed.

Large droplet nuclei particle size is >5μ in diameter containing infectious particles. These droplets do not remain suspended in the air long and travel only short distances. Transmission from larger droplets requires close contact (ie within 3 feet) between the infected source and the recipient. Examples of diseases caused by large droplet nuclei are meningococcal meningitis, pertussis, streptococcal pharyngitis, multidrug resistant *Strep.pneumoniae* etc.

Location	A single room with a wash hand basin and preferably with an en suite toilet.
	The door must be kept closed at all times except for necessary entrances and exits.
	Remove any unnecessary furniture before admitting the patient.
	Ensure that there is an adequate supply of hand wash antiseptic/detergent preparation and disposable paper towels.
	Ensure that there is a clinical waste bin with a yellow plastic bag inside the room.
Staff	Only staff who have immunity against varicella and measles should care for these patients and their number should be restricted, if possible. Refer to page 98 for patient with pulmonary tuberculosis.
Visitors	All visitors must seek advice from the nurse–in–charge of the ward before visiting patient.
Protective clothing	*Gloves:* Not usually necessary, but should be worn only for contact with respiratory secretions or contact with contaminated articles.
	Plastic Aprons/gowns: Not usually necessary, but should be worn for contact with the patients and their environment to prevent contamination of clothing.
	Masks: Wear mask when entering the room of a patient with known or suspected tuberculosis.
	Eye Protection: Not necessary.

Hand hygiene	Wash hands thoroughly with an antiseptic/detergent and dry with a disposable paper towel. Hands must be washed after touching the patient or potentially contaminated articles and before taking care of another patient.
Laundry	Processed as infected linen according to the local policy.
Equipment	Single-use disposable respiratory equipment and accessories should be used where possible. If items of equipment are re-used then they should be thoroughly cleaned and disinfected or sterilized.
Decontamination & waste disposal	Any equipment which may be soiled with respiratory secretions should be decontaminated by thorough cleaning and disinfected or sterilized.
	Waste: All waste, including items contaminated with respiratory secretions must be discarded into a clinical waste bag.
CSSD	Respiratory equipment must be cleaned, and heat disinfected preferably in CSSD. Inform the CSSD manager of the infection risk from the equipment.
Body fluid spills	Any spillage or gross contamination by respiratory secretions must be cleaned immediately using disposable cloths. It must be disinfected and cleaned according to local policy.
Inter-departmental visits	Limit the movement and transport of the patient to essential purposes only. Seek advice from member of Infection Control Team.
Laboratory specimens	If pulmonary tuberculosis is suspected, or confirmed record this on the request form and label sputum specimen, and request form with a "Danger of Infection - Take special care" label.
Last offices	The infection control precautions employed during life must be continued after death.
	In the case of open tuberculosis, the body must be conspicuously labelled with a "Danger of Infection" label on the wrist, the wrapping sheet or shroud and on the information sheet.

CONTACT ISOLATION

These precautions are used for patients to prevent the transmission of communicable diseases and epidemiologically important microorganisms which are causing infection or colonization and which are transmitted by direct patient contact or indirectly by contact with the patient or the patient's, environment, excretion and secretion. Examples of these infections include gonococcal conjunctivitis of newborn, disseminated herpes simplex, streptococcal & staphylococcal infections, methicillin-resistant *Staph. aureus* (MRSA), multi-resistant Gram-negative bacteria, vancomycin resistant enterococci (VRE).

Location A single room with an en suite toilet is necessary if the infective agent be disseminated into the environment or when the microorganism is particularly resistant.

Staff Usually none except if they are caring for a patient with MRSA, in which case health care workers with skin conditions should be excluded.

Visitors Visitors must always report to the sister or nurse-in-charge before entering the room.

Protective clothing *Gloves:* Wear close fitting non-sterile single-use disposable gloves for contact with the infected site, dressing and secretions.

Plastic Aprons: Wear a disposable plastic apron for the delivery of direct care. Discard into a clinical waste bin after use.

Gowns: Use only for extensive physical contact when gross soiling is likely.

Masks: Usually not necessary but recommended for patients with MRSA for procedures that may generate Staphylococcal aerosols (see page 86).

Eye Protection: Not necessary.

Hand hygiene Hands must be washed thoroughly with an antiseptic/detergent preparation and dried using disposable paper towels. They should be washed after contact with the patient or contaminated articles and before taking care of another patient.

Equipment Articles contaminated with infective material should be discarded if they are single-use disposable, or cleaned and disinfected preferably in CSSD.

Laundry	Is processed as infected linen according to the local policy.
Decontamination & waste disposal	*CSSD:* Non-disposable items should be sent to CSSD for disinfection/sterilization. *Waste:* Contaminated waste is disposed of as clinical waste according to local policy.
Body fluid spills	Disinfect and clean the spills from infected secretions as outlined in the disinfection policy.
Inter-departmental visits	Seek advice from the Infection Control Nurse.

ENTERIC ISOLATION

For those infections which are spread by the faecal-oral route. Examples include all microorganisms causing gastroenteritis eg *Salmonella, Shigella, Clostridium difficile*, viral causes of diarrhoea and hepatitis A & E. The patient should be nursed in a single room with an en suite toilet facilities.

All patients with enteric infection should be requested to wash their hands with soap under running water after using the toilet. In the paediatric ward, parents and staff should be reminded to wash and dry their hands thoroughly after changing a baby's nappy.

Location	A single room with a wash hand basin and an en suite toilet.
	Check that an adequate supply of toilet tissue is provided in the toilet area.
	Check that an adequate supply of hand cleanser and paper towels are supplied at the wash hand basin.
Staff	No exclusions.
Visitors	Visitors must report to the sister or nurse-in-charge before entering the room for instructions regarding the infection control measures.
Protective clothing	*Gloves:* Are worn for contact with faecal material or any item likely to be contaminated with infective material.
	Plastic Aprons: Are worn for delivery of direct patients care, or for contact with faecal material or items likely to be contaminated with the infective material.

Gowns: Are required only if extensive soiling with faecal material is likely.

Masks: Not necessary.

Eye Protection: Not necessary.

Hand hygiene

Hands must be washed thoroughly with antiseptic/detergent preparation and dried with a disposable paper towel after contact with the patient, contaminated articles, after removing gloves, and before taking care of another patient.

Equipment

When bedpans or commodes are used, these must be reserved for the patient's exclusive use. These must be decontaminated after each use and only returned to communal use after terminal disinfection by heat or using an appropriate chemical disinfectant.

Alternatively, disposable bedpans may be used. These must be disposed of into a macerator unit.

Other items or equipment which may have faecal contamination must be decontaminated by thorough cleaning and disinfected either by heat or chemical disinfectant depending upon the item to be disinfected.

Decontamination & waste disposal

CSSD: No specific precautions
Waste: All waste which is contaminated with faecal material must be disposed of as clinical waste.

Spillage of faecal material

Spillage of faecal material should be cleaned immediately using disposable cloths or wipes and disinfected with an appropriate chemical disinfectant. Seek advice from the Infection Control Nurse.

BLOOD AND BODY FLUIDS ISOLATION

For those infections which are spread by blood and body fluids. Examples include infection by blood-borne viruses (hepatitis B, C, HIV infection etc). Isolation of the patient is not necessary unless they are bleeding or likely to bleed, have diarrhoea or other infections. Patients with healing wounds, those who have open lesions or a drain inserted, those who are unconscious, uncooperative, mentally abnormal and those who are fitting should be nursed in a single room.

Location	Isolation of patient in a single ward is usually not necessary (see above).
Staff	All cuts, abrasions or broken skin must be covered with a waterproof dressing.
	Exclude staff who have extensive areas of broken skin, which may not be adequately covered with a waterproof dressing. These staff should seek advice from the Occupational Health Department.
Visitors	If the patient is in the isolation room, the visitor must report to the nurse-in-charge before entering the room.
Protective clothing	*Gloves:* Must be worn in situations where soiling of blood or body fluids exposure is likely.
	Plastic Aprons: Must be worn for any activity where blood or body fluid exposure is anticipated.
	Gowns: Impervious or water repellant single-use disposable gown with long sleeves and fitted cuff must be worn in any situation where there is a likelihood of splashing of blood or body fluids.
	Masks: Must be worn in situations where splashing of blood or body fluids is likely.
	Eye Protection: Must be worn when blood or body fluids splashes are likely.
	Other: Full length plastic aprons and rubber boots may be required to protect the legs and feet during invasive procedures likely to generate extensive dissemination of blood or body fluids.
Hand hygiene	Hands must be washed thoroughly with an antiseptic/detergent preparation and dried using disposable paper towels. They should be washed immediately if contaminated with blood or body fluids, after removing protective clothing, ie gloves, plastic apron etc, and before taking care of another patient.
Equipment	Any re-usable equipment which has been contaminated with blood or body fluids must be thoroughly cleaned and disinfected by heat or by using a suitable virucidal agent.

Laundry

All linen must be processed as infected linen according to the local policy.

Decontamination & waste disposal

CSSD: All CSSD items must be placed inside a clear plastic bag, sealed and transported in an appropriate rigid container. The CSSD manager must be informed that the equipment was used on a high risk patient. The equipment must only be cleaned in the CSSD by trained staff wearing appropriate protective clothing.

Any equipment contaminated with blood or body fluids should be decontaminated by thorough cleaning followed by either heat or chemical disinfectant as specified in the local disinfection policy.

Waste: All waste which is contaminated with blood or body fluids must be disposed of as clinical waste according to the local policy.

Body fluid spill

Spillage of blood and certain other body fluids must be disinfected and cleaned using chlorine-based disinfectant as outlined on page 70.

Inter-departmental visits

No restrictions provided that the appropriate infection control precautions are maintained.

Laboratory specimens

Laboratory specimens from the patient must not be collected by untrained medical students, inexperienced phlebotomist etc. They must be handled carefully, ensuring that the outside of the container is not contaminated. They must also be correctly labelled and packaged, ie the request form must be kept separate from the specimen in a plastic bag. Specimens must have a "Danger of Infection – Take special care" label both on the request form and on the specimen. All specimens must be transported to the laboratory in an appropriate container.

Last offices

The infection control precautions employed during life must be continued after death. All bleeding points must be covered with a secure occlusive dressing. All relevant personnel should be notified about the danger of infection.

The body must be transported in a cadaver bag and must be labelled with a "Danger of Infection" sticker on the identity band on the wrapping sheet or shroud and on the outside of the cadaver bag.

Only minimal handling of the body by trained personnel is permissible. The body *must not* be embalmed.

PROTECTIVE ISOLATION

Protective isolation is used for severely immunocompromised patients who are highly susceptible and need protection from infection from persons and the environment. It is important that all immunocompromised patients should be kept separate from other patients who are infected or have conditions that make infection transmission more likely.

Isolation measures are usually maximum for patients undergoing transplantation. Most infections acquired by the immunosuppressed patients are endogenous in origin and isolation in a single room is of doubtful value. However if the side rooms are required for protection, it should be under positive pressure ventilation.

Location	A single room with a wash hand basin and with en suite toilet facilities.
	The room and equipment must be cleaned before the patient enters.
Staff	Staff who have or may have an infectious condition must not attend patients in this category.
Visitors	Exclude visitors who have, or may have an infectious condition.
Protective clothing	*Gloves:* Not necessary.
	Plastic Aprons: Disposable plastic aprons should be worn by staff delivering direct patient care.
	Gowns: Not necessary.
	Masks: Not necessary.
	Eye Protection: Not necessary.
Hand hygiene	Hands must be washed thoroughly and dried with disposable paper towels before and after contact with the patient.

Equipment It may be necessary to disinfect some items of equipment before use. Please consult a member of the Infection Control Team for advice.

Inter-departmental visits Should be arranged so that the patient is seen immediately to avoid contact with other patients who may have infectious conditions.

Table 2.1 – Isolation and infection control precautions for infectious diseases and epidemiologically important microorganisms.

Disease	Category of isolation and precautions	Duration of infection controls precautions	Comments
Acquired Immune Deficiency Syndrome (AIDS)	Blood & Body Fluids		See Chapter 5 for details.
Actinomycosis	None		
Amoebiasis			
Dysentery	Enteric	As long as cysts appear in faeces.	—
Liver abscess	None	—	—
Anthrax			
Cutaneous	Contact	Duration of hospitalization. (Until off antibiotics and cultures are negative).	• Inform ICD and notify CCDC. • Contact microbiologist and laboratory must be informed of any specimens sent for examination.
Pulmonary (or systemic)	Strict	Duration of hospitalization. (Until off antibiotics and cultures are negative).	—
Ascariasis	None	—	—
Aspergillosis	None	—	—
Botulism	None	—	—
Brucellosis	Contact	Precautions only if draining lesion(s).	Person-to-person transmission rare.
Campylobacter gastroenteritis	Enteric	Duration of diarrhoea.	Not usually transmitted from person-to-person.
Candidiasis	Contact	Duration of illness.	Spread rare, except in high dependency units, ie SCBU, ICU etc.
Cat-scratch fever	None	—	—
Chancroid	None	—	—

Table 2.1 – *continued*

Disease	Category of isolation and precautions	Duration of infection control precautions	Comments
Chickenpox (Varicella)	Respiratory & Contact	Exclusion should continue until lesions are crusted. (Patient is Infectious from 2 days before until 5 days after rash appears)	See page 104 for details. • Discharge patient home if clinical condition permits. • Health care workers should have a clear history of chickenpox or should know that they are immune. • Visitors who have not had the disease must be warned of the risk.
Chlamydia trachomatis infection			
Conjunctivitis	Contact	Duration of symptoms.	—
Genital	Contact	Duration of symptoms.	—
Respiratory	Respiratory	Duration of illness.	—
Cholera	Enteric	Duration of illness	• Inform ICD and notify CCDC. • Until 3 cultures of stools are negative.
Clostridium perfringens			
Food Poisoning	None	—	—
Gas Gangrene	Contact	Duration of illness.	• Usually autogenous infection. • Not transmitted from person-to-person. • Isolation of patient not necessary.
Clostridium difficile	Enteric	Duration of diarrhoea.	See page 107 for detail.
Conjunctivitis			
Gonococcal	Contact	Until 24 hours after starting antibiotic therapy.	—
Cryptococcus	None	—	—
Cryptosporidiosis	Enteric	Duration of diarrhoea.	—

Table 2.1 – *continued*

Disease	Category of isolation and precautions	Duration of infection control precautions	Comments
Cytomegalovirus	Usually none	—	Pregnant staff should avoid contact, particularly with patient's urine.
Diarrhoea	Enteric	—	See page 96 for details.
Diphtheria			
Cutaneous	Strict	Until off antibiotics and 3 swabs are culture negative from skin lesions taken at least 24 hours apart after antibiotic therapy.	• Throat and nasal swabs should be taken from all close contacts. • Notify laboratory and microbiologist before swabbing contacts. • Inform ICD and notify CCDC.
Pharyngeal	Strict	Until off antibiotics and 3 consecutive swabs from nose and throat are culture negative.	• Culture positive carriers of toxigenic *Corynebacterium diphtheria* should receive chemoprophylaxis with erythromycin and swabs repeated after treatment as advised by the ICD. • No admission of patients until contacts are bacteriologically clear. • Inform ICD and notify CCDC.
Dysentry			
Amoebic	Enteric	As long as cysts appear in faeces.	—
Bacillary	Enteric	Until 3 cultures of stools are negative.	Discharge patient home if clinical condition permits.
Echinococcosis (Hydatidosis)	None	—	—
Ebola virus	Strict	During hospitalisation.	See page 117 for details.
Encephalitis or encephalomyelitis	Respiratory and Enteric	4 days to several weeks according to causative organism.	Consult member of ICT for advice.
Erysipelas	Contact	Until off antibiotic and cultures are negative.	—

Table 2.1 – *continued*

Disease	Category of isolation and precautions	Duration of infection control precautions	Comments
Enteric fever			
Typhoid	Enteric	6-12 consecutive culture negative stools.	• Inform ICD and notify CCDC.
Paratyphoid	Enteric	6-12 consecutive culture negative stools.	—
Epiglottis (*H.Influenzae* type b)	Respiratory	—	• Inform ICD and notify CCDC. • Close contacts should be given rifampicin as chemoprophylaxis at the advice of CCDC.
Gas Gangrene	Contact	Duration of illness.	• Usually autogenous infection. • Not transmitted from person-to-person. • Isolation of patient not necessary.
Gastroenteritis	Enteric	—	See page 96 for details.
Glandular fever	Oral secretions precautions.	Until acute phase is over.	Isolation of patient not necessary
German Measles (Rubella)	Respiratory	From 7 days before up to 10 days from onset of rash.	• Discharge patient home if clinical condition permits. • Exclude non-immune women (staff or visitor) of child bearing age.
Gonococcal			
Ophthalmia neonatorum	Contact	For 24 hours after the start of effective antibiotic therapy.	—
Gonorrhoea	Contact	Until culture negative ie 24 hrs after effective antibiotic therapy.	—
Granulocytopenia	Protective	At the direction of the clinician.	Consult member of ICT for advice.

Table 2.1 – continued

Disease	Category of isolation and precautions	Duration of infection control precautions	Comments
Hepatitis, viral			
Type A	Enteric	7 days before to 7 days after onset of jaundice.	• Hepatitis A is most contagious before jaundice and is infectious in the early febrile phase of illness. • Close contacts may be given gamma globulin within 14 days to abort or attenuate clinical illness.
Type B	Blood & Body Fluids	—	See page 131 for details.
Type C	Blood & Body Fluids	—	See page 134 for details.
Type E	Enteric	Duration of diarrhoea.	—
Herpes simplex (including congenital herpes)	Contact	Until vesicles healed.	• Protect immunologically compromised patients. • Wear gloves when hands are in contact with oral or genital secretions. • Staff with cold sores should not work with compromised patients, neonates or burns patients.
Herpes zoster (Shingles)	Contact	Length of acute illness ie until vesicles dry.	• As herpes zoster may lead to cases of chicken-pox, susceptible individuals and staff who have not had chickenpox must be excluded from contact with the patient. • Visitors who have not had chickenpox should be warned of the risks.
HIV Human Immuno-deficiency Virus)	Blood & Body Fluids	—	• Isolation required in special circumstances. • See page 28 and 135 for details.
Hookworm disease	None	—	—

Table 2.1 – *continued*

Disease	Category of isolation and precautions	Duration of infection control precautions	Comments
Immuno-compromised status	Protective	At the discretion of the clinician.	Seek advice from the ICD. See page 31 for details.
Impetigo	Contact	For 24 hours after start of effective antibiotic therapy.	—
Infectious mononucleosis (Glandular fever)	None	Until acute phase is over.	Oral secretions precautions.
Influenza	Respiratory	In prodromal phase and for 5 days after onset.	Immunization can be offered to a selected group.
Lassa fever	Strict	Duration of hospitalization.	See page 117 for details.
Legionnaire's disease	None	—	• Inform ICD and notify CCDC. • Not transmitted from person-to-person. • Isolation of patient not necessary. • See page 110 for details.
Leprosy	None	—	—
Leptospirosis (Weil's disease)	None	Duration of hospitalization.	• Contact precautions for urine only. • Not transmitted from person-to-person. • Isolation of patient not necessary.
Listeriosis	Contact	Duration of hospitalization.	• Person-to-person spread rare. • Isolate neonates and mothers only.
Lyme disease	None	—	—
Malaria	None	—	—
Marburg virus disease	Strict	Duration of hospitalization.	See page 117 for details.

Table 2.1 – *continued*

Disease	Category of isolation and precautions	Duration of infection control precautions	Comments
Measles	Respiratory	For 5 days after start of rash, except in immunocompromised patients with whom precautions should be maintained for duration of illness.	• Discharge patient home if clinical condition permits. • Immunoglobulin for exposed immuno-compromised patient • If outbreak in paediatric ward, do not admit children who are not immune until 14 days after the last contact has gone home.
Meningitis			
"Coliforms"	None	—	—
Listeria monocytogenes	None	—	See under Listeriosis.
Neisseria meningitidis (Meningococcal)	Respiratory	For 48 hours after start of effective antibiotic therapy and patient has received chemoprophylaxis.	• Visiting by all children should be discontinued. • Inform ICD and notify CCDC. • See page 90 for details.
Haemophilus influenzae (type b)	Respiratory	Duration of illness.	Close contacts should be given rifampicin as prophylaxis at the advice of CCDC.
Pneumococcal Meningitis	None	—	—
Tuberculous Meningitis	None or Respiratory	—	• Isolate if patient has respiratory open pulmonary tuberculosis. • See page 98 for details.
Viral	Respiratory & Enteric	Until virus no longer present in stool.	Seek advice from a member of ICT.
Meningococcal septicaemia	Respiratory	For 48 hours after start of effective antibiotic therapy and patient has received chemoprophylaxis.	See page 90 for details.

Table 2.1 – *continued*

Disease	Category of isolation and precautions	Duration of infection control precautions	Comments
MRSA (Methicillin Resistant *Staph. aureus*)	Contact	Until 3 swabs are negative.	See page 83 for details.
Multi-resistant Gram- negative organisms	Contact	—	• Seek advice from a member of ICT. • See page 114 for details.
Mumps	Respiratory	7 days before to 9 days after onset of parotid swelling.	• Exclude non-immune staff. • Inform visitors who are not immune. • Persons with subclinical infection may be infectious.
Mycoplasma	None	—	—
Norcadia	None	—	—
Orf	None or contact	—	• Contact precautions for exudate. • Isolation of patient not necessary.
Pertussis (see Whooping cough)	—	—	—
Pinworm infection	None	—	—
Plague			
Bubonic	Strict	Duration of hospitalization until culture negative.	Inform ICD and notify CCDC.
Pneumonia	Strict	Duration of hospitalization until culture negative.	Inform ICD and notify CCDC.
Pneumonia	Usually none (see comments)	—	Isolation required with respiratory precautions for *Strep. pneumonia* resistant to penicillin, MRSA, plague and psittacosis.

Table 2.1 – *continued*

Disease	Category of isolation and precautions	Duration of infection control precautions	Comments
Poliomyelitis	Respiratory and Enteric	Until stools negative for polio virus or 7 days from onset.	• Droplet spread is possible during the earliest phase first week); masks should be worn. Subsequently, faecal excretion is more important. • Visitors and staff should be immunized. • Gamma globulin for non-immune contacts, booster for immunized contacts. • No elective surgery on non-immunized contacts. • Virus shedding may follow vaccination with a live oral polio vaccine for several weeks.
Psittacosis (Q fever)	Respiratory	For 7 days after onset.	Inform ICD and notify CCDC.
Rabies	Contact	Duration of hospitalization.	• Inform ICD and notify CCDC. • Immunize staff in close contact. • See page 121 for details.
Ringworm	Contact	—	Isolation in a cubicle is advisable especially in Paediatric ward.
Rubella	Respiratory	From 7 days before up to 10 days from onset of rash.	• Discharge patient home if clinical condition permits. • Exclude non-immune women (staff or visitor) of child bearing age.
Salmonellosis (not typhoid or paratyphoid)	Enteric	Duration of diarrhoea.	• Staff (except in catering or food handler) may return to work at the advice of the OHD when free of symptoms (ie formed stool) but should not handle drugs or food until culture negative. • See page 96 for details.

Table 2.1 – *continued*

Disease	Category of isolation and precautions	Duration of infection control precautions	Comments
Scabies	Contact	Until completion of appropriate treatment.	See page 128 for details.
Schistosomiasis (Biliharziasis)	None	—	—
Shigellosis	Enteric	Until 3 cultures of stools are negative.	—
Streptococci β Haemolytic			
Group A (*Strep. pyogenes*)	Contact	Until off antibiotics and cultures are negative.	—
Group B	Usually none	—	Cross-infection can occur in SCBU, seek advice from member of ICT.
Group C	Usually none	—	—
Group G	Usually none	—	—
Staphylococcal (food poisoning)	None	—	—
Syphilis			
Congenital, primary and secondary	Contact	For 48 hours after start of effective therapy.	Skin lesions of primary and secondary syphilis may be highly infectious.
Latent (tertiary) and seropositive without lesions	None	—	
Tetanus	None	—	—
Thread worm	None	—	—
Toxocara	None	—	—
Toxoplasmosis	None	—	—
Trichomoniasis	None	—	—
Trichuriasis (Whipworm)	None	—	—

Table 2.1 – *continued*

Disease	Category of isolation and precautions	Duration of infection control precautions	Comments
Tuberculosis			
Pulmonary (open)	Respiratory	- Two weeks after start of effective antimicrobial treatment and sputum is negative for AAFB. - Four weeks in neonatal and paediatric wards or if immunosuppressed patients are present.	• Inform ICD and notify CCDC. • Staff and visitors who are not immune should be warned of the risk and given suitable protection ie face mask. • See page 98 for details.
Closed	None	—	• All suspected cases should be notified to CCDC. • Isolation of patient not necessary.
Typhoid/ Paratyphoid fever	Enteric	Until 6 -12 consecutive stools are negative and urine if applicable.	• Inform ICD and notify CCDC.
Vincent's angina (Trench mouth)	None	—	—
Viral Haemorrhagic Fevers	Strict	Duration of hospitalization.	See page 117 for details.
VRE (Vancomycin resistant enterococci)	Contact	—	See page 115 for details.
Whooping cough (Pertussis)	Respiratory	Until 3 weeks after onset of paroxysmal cough or 7 days after start of effective antibiotic therapy.	• Discharge patient home if clinical condition permits. • Visiting by children should be restricted to those who are immune. • Prophylactic erythromycin to close contacts as advised by the ICD.

Table 2.1 – *continued*

Disease	Category of isolation and precautions	Dration of infection controls precautions	Comments
Wound infections			
Major/extensive or *Strep. pyogenes*, MRSA, multi-resistant organisms.	Contact	Until negative cultures.	—
Minor	None	—	—
Yellow fever	None	—	—

References and further reading

Ayliffe GAJ, Lowbury EJL, Geddes AM, Williams JD. Prevention of Infection in Ward II: Isolation of patients. In: *Control of Hospital Infection - A practical handbook*. 3rd ed. London: Chapman & Hall, 1992: 142-169.

Garner JS. Guidelines for isolation precautions in hospitals. *American Journal of Infection Control* 1996; **24**: 24-52.

Bennson AS, ed. *Control of Communicable Diseases Manual*. 16th ed. Washington: American Public Health Association, 1995.

Bagshawe KD, Blowers R, Lidwell OM. Isolating patients in hospital to control infection. *British Medical Journal* 1978; **2**: 609-612, 684-686, 744-748, 808-811, 879-881.

Rahman M. Commissioning a new hospital isolation unit and assessment of its use over five years. *Journal of Hospital Infection* 1985; **6**: 65-70.

Breuer J, Jeffries DJ. Control of viral infections in hospitals. *Journal of Hospital Infection* 1990; **16**: 191-221.

Goldmann DA. The role of barrier precautions in infection. *Journal of Hospital Infection* 1991; **18** (Supplement A): 515-523.

Patterson JE. Isolation of Patients with Communicable Disease. In: Mayhall CG, ed. *Hospital Epidemiology and Infection Control*. Baltimore: Williams & Wilkins, 1996; 1032-1051.

Beekman SE, Henderson DK. Controversies in Isolation Policies and Practices. In: Wenzel RP, ed. *Prevention and Control of Nosocomical Infections*. 3rd ed. Balitmore: Williams & Wilkins 1997: 71-84.

APPENDIX I

LIST OF NOTIFIABLE DISEASES IN THE UNITED KINGDOM

England and Wales

Acute encephalitis	Measles	Scarlet fever
Acute poliomyelitis	Meningitis	Smallpox
Anthrax	Meningococcal septicaemia	Tetanus
Cholera	(without meningitis)	Tuberculosis
Dysentery	Mumps	Typhoid fever
Diphtheria	Ophthalmia neonatorum	Typhus
(amoebic or bacillary)	Paratyphoid fever	Viral haemorrhagic
Food poisoning	Plague	fevers
Leprosy	Rabies	Viral hepatitis
Leptospirosis	Relapsing fever	Whooping cough
Malaria	Rubella	Yellow fever

Notifiable to the Local Authority's 'proper' officer which is usually the Consultant in Communicable Disease Control.

Scotland

Anthrax	Measles	Smallpox
Bacillary dysentery	Meningococcal	Tetanus
Chickenpox	infection	Toxoplasmosis
Cholera	Mumps	Tuberculosis
Diphtheria	Paratyphoid	(respiratory &
Erysipelas	Plague	non-respiratory)
Food poisoning	Poliomyelitis	Typhoid fever
Legionellosis	Puerperal fever	Typhus fever
Leptospirosis	Rabies	Viral haemorrhagic
Lyme disease	Relapsing fever	fevers
Malaria	Rubella	Viral hepatitis
	Scarlet fever	Whooping cough

Notifiable to Director of Public Health or Consultant in Public Health in the appropriate Health Board.

Northern Ireland

Acute encephalitis/
  meningitis: bacterial
Acute encephalitis/
  meningitis: viral
Anthrax
Chickenpox
Cholera
Diphtheria
Dysentery
Food Poisoning
Gastroenteritis
  (under 2 years of age only)
Hepatitis A

Hepatitis B
Hepatitis unspecified:
  viral
Legionnaire's disease
Leptospirosis
Malaria
Measles
Mumps
Paratyphoid fever
Plague
Poliomyelitis: acute
Rabies
Relapsing fever

Rubella
Scarlet fever
Smallpox
Tetanus
Tuberculosis
  (pulmonary and
  non-pulmonary)
Typhoid fever
Typhus
Viral haemorrhagic
  fevers
Whooping cough
Yellow fever

Notifiable to the Director of Public Health or Consultant in Communicable Disease Control of the appropriate Health and Social Service Board.

Notification of AIDS

AIDS is not a notifiable disease, but doctors are urged to report in a voluntary confidential scheme. AIDS cases should be reported on a special AIDS form in strict medical confidence to the Director, Public Health Laboratory Service, Communicable Disease Surveillance Centre (CDSC), 61 Colindale Avenue, London, NW9 5EQ. Advice about the reporting of cases may be obtained from CDSC (Tel: 0181 200 6868), or locally from the CCDC or genito-urinary physicians.

Cases of HIV infection and AIDS seen by paediatricians are reported through the British Paediatric Association Surveillance Unit, while in pregnant women they are reported through the Royal College of Obstetricians and Gynaecologists Survey of HIV in Pregnancy. Reports of both are received by the Department of Epidemiology, Institute of Child Health, Guilford Street, London WC1N 1EH (Tel: 0171 829 8686). All reporting is voluntary and confidential.

APPENDIX II

Incubation Periods

Diseases	*Average Period (range)*
AIDS/HIV	variable – may be years
Amoebic dysentry	2-4 weeks (few days to several months)
Anthrax	A few hours to 7 days (most cases occur within 48 hours after exposure)
Ascariasis	4-8 weeks
Aspergillosis	unknown
Botulism	12-36 hours (up to several days) (Infant botulism 3 days to 2 weeks)
Brucellosis	5-60 days (highly variable may be up to several months)
Campylobacter enteritis	3-5 days (1-10 days)
Candidiasis	2-5 days
Cat-scratch disease	3-10 days to appearance of primary lesion, further 2-6 weeks to appearance of lymphadenopathy
Chancroid (*H.ducreyi*)	3-5 days (up to 14 days)
Chickenpox (Varicella)	13-17 days (10-21 days ; may be prolonged after passive immunization against varicella and in the immunodeficient)
Chlamydial conjunctivitis (*Chlamydia trachomatis*)	5-12 days (3 days-6 weeks in newborns; 6-19 days in adult)
Cytomegalovirus (CMV)	Within 3-8 weeks after transplant or transfusion with infected blood; infection acquired during first birth is demonstrable 3-12 weeks in newborn after delivery
Dengue Fever	7-10 days (3-14 days)
Dermatophytoses	See *under* Tinea
Diphtheria	2-5 days (2-7 days)
Erytherma infectiosum (Fifth disease or parvovirus)	4-10 days (variable)
Gastroenteritis (viral)	
Adenovirus	8-10 days
Astrovirus	1-2 days
Calcivirus	1-3 days
Norwalk	12-48 hours
Rotavirus	1-3 days

Continued over the page

Diseases	Average Period (range)
Gastroenteritis & food poisoning (bacterial)	
Salmonellosis	12–36 hours (6–72 hours)
Shigellosis (Bacillary dysentry)	1–3 days (12–96 hours)
Campylobacter jejuni/coli	3–5 days (1–10 days)
Staphylococcus aureus	2–4 hours (30 min to 7 hours)
Clostridium difficile	5–10 days (few days to 8 weeks) after stopping antibiotics
Clostridium perfringens	10–12 hours (6–24 hours)
Clostridium botulinum	12–36 hours (12–96 hours)
Cryptosporidiosis	7 days (2–14 days)
Giardiasis (*Giardia lamblia*)	7–10 days (5–25 days)
Bacillus cereus	1–6 hours where vomiting is predominant symptom 6–24 hours where diarrhoea is predominant
Cholera	1–3 days (few hours to 5 days)
Escherichia coli (Entero-invasive [EIEC])	10–18 hours
Escherichia coli (Enteropathogenic [EPEC])	9–12 hours (probably)
Escherichia coli (Enterotoxigenic [ETEC])	1–5 days
Escherichia coli 0157:H7 (Verocyotoxin [VTEC])	1–3 days (12–60 hours)
Vibrio parahaemolyticus	12–24 hours (2–96 hours)
Yersinia enterocolitica	24–36 hours (3–7 days)
Aeromonas hydrophila	12–48 hours
Listeria monocytogenes	48 hours – 7 weeks
Gonorrhoea	2–7 days genito-urinary; 1–5days ophthalmia neonatorum
***Haemophilus influenzae* type b infection**	2–4 days (probably)
Hand, foot and mouth disease	3–5 days
Hepatitis	
Hepatitis A	25–30 days (15–50 days)
Hepatitis B	75 days (45–180 days)
Hepatitis C	20 days–13 weeks (2 weeks – 6 months)
Hepatatis D	35 days (2–8weeks)
Hepatitis E	15–64 days (26–42 days)
Herpes simplex	2–14 days (2–28 days perinatal infection)
Impetigo	
Streptococcal	7–10 days
Staphylococcal	1–10 days

Continued over the page

Diseases	Average Period (range)
Infectious mononucleosis (Glandular fever)	4-6 weeks
Influenza	1-5 days
Legionnaires' disease	5-6 days (2-10 days for pneumonia);1-2 days for pontaic fever
Leishmaniasis	
Visceral	few weeks to 6 months
Cutaneous	few weeks
Leptospirosis	10 days (4-19 days)
Listeriosis	3 days to 10 weeks
Lyme disease	7-10 days (3-32 days) after tick exposure
Lymphocytic choriomeningitis	8-13 days (15-21 days)
Lymphogranuloma venereum	3-30 days
Malaria	
P. falciparum	7-14 days
P. vivax	8-14 days
P. ovale	8-14 days
P. malariae	7-30 days
Measles	8-12 days (7-18 days)
Meningococcal disease	3-4 days (2-10 days)
Molluscum contagiosum	2-7 weeks (7 days to 6 months)
Mumps	16-18 days (12-25 days)
Mycoplasma pneumoniae	6-23 days
Pertussis (Whooping cough)	7-10 days (6-20 days)
Plague	
Bubonic	2-6 days
Pneumonic	2-4 days
Pneumocystis carinii	Unknown
Poliomyelitis	7-14 days (3-35 days)
Psittacosis (*Chlamydia psittaci*)	1-4 weeks
Q fever (*Coxiella burnetii*)	2-3 weeks (depends on size of infecting dose)
Rabies	2-8 weeks (5 days to a year or more, depends on the site and severity of the wound; injury closer to brain has shorter incubation period)

Continued over the page

Diseases	*Average Period (range)*
Relapsing fever (*B. recurrentis*)	8 days (5-15 days)
Respiratory syncytial virus	4-6 days (2-8 days)
Ringworm	
Tinea capitis (scalp ringworm)	10-14 days
Tinea corporis (body ringworm)	4-10 days
Tinea pedis (athlete's foot)	Unknown
Tinea unguim	Unknown
Roseola infantum	8-10 days
Rubella (German measles)	16-18 days (14-32 days)
Salmonellosis	12-36 hours (6 hours -3days)
Scabies	2-6 weeks without previous exposure; 1-4 days re-infection
Shigellosis	1-3 days (12-96 hours)
Syphilis	3 weeks (10 days to 3 months)
Tetanus	3-21 days (1 day to several months depending upon the character, extent and the location of wound)
Threadworms	Unknown
Toxic shock syndrome	2 days
Toxocariasis	Weeks to several months depending on the intensity of infection. Up to 10 years for ocular symptoms
Toxoplasmosis	7 days (4-21 days)
Tuberculosis	4-12 weeks (variable)
Typhoid & paratyphoid fevers	1-3 weeks (3-60 days)
Typhus fever	12 days (1-2 weeks)
Viral haemorrhagic fevers	
Marburg	3-9 days
Ebola	2-21 days
Lassa	6-21 days
Yellow fever	3-6 days

3

DISINFECTION POLICY

Medical and surgical devices may serve as a vehicles for transmission of infectious diseases to susceptible hosts. Therefore it is important that all hospitals and health care facilities should a have a disinfection policy. The aim of a disinfection policy is to remove visible soil/dirt and invisible microorganisms making patients' items/equipment safe to prevent cross-infection between patients and to protect personnel from the infected items and equipment.

METHODS OF DECONTAMINATION

It is important to have a clear understanding of the terms and classification used in this process and to choose the most appropriate procedure for the items or surfaces in question.

Cleaning is a process which removes soil, eg dust, dirt and organic matter, along with a large proportion of microorganisms; a further reduction will occur on drying, as microorganisms cannot multiply on a clean dry surface. Thorough cleaning with soap/detergent and water is adequate for most surfaces in the hospital environment and is a *prerequisite* before disinfection and sterilization is commenced.

Disinfection by either heat or chemicals will destroy microorganisms but not bacterial spores. Chemical disinfection does not necessarily kill all microorganisms present but reduces them to a level not harmful to health. Chemical disinfection should only be used if heat treatment is impractical or may cause damage to the equipment. Chemical disinfectants are classified as chemical sterilants used to disinfect heat sensitive items if they can kill bacterial spores (which normally require prolonged exposure time); This process may be more accurately described as *high level* disinfection. Disinfectants are used on inanimate objects only and not on living tissue. Chemicals used to kill microorganisms on skin or living tissue are known as **antiseptics**.

Sterilization is a process which achieves the complete destruction or removal of all microorganisms, including bacterial spores. Equipment and materials used in procedures involving a break in the skin or mucous membranes should be sterilized, eg surgical instruments and products intended for parenteral use or for instillation into sterile body cavities.

If the sterilization is not carried out in the hospital CSSD then it is vital that sterilization procedures outside a central processing department promote the same level of safety and efficiency. Requirements include routine biological, mechanical and chemical monitoring to ensure that all parameters of sterilization are met before using the instrument on or in a patient.

The choice of method of disinfection or sterilization depends mainly on type of material to be disinfected, level of decontamination required for the procedure and microorganisms involved.

The outcome of a disinfection procedure is affected by the presence of organic load (bioburden) on the item, type and level of microbial contaminant, prior cleaning of the object, disinfection concentration and exposure time, physical structure of the object and temperature and pH of the disinfection process.

RISKS OF INFECTION FROM EQUIPMENT

The risks of infection from equipment may be classified into four categories (see below) and placing instruments and equipment in one of the following categories assists in choosing the proper level of disinfection or sterilization needed to protect the patients and the health care worker.

Pre-cleaning of instruments before further decontamination is an essential procedure. This allows physical removal of microorganisms which prevents inactivation of the disinfectant by organic matter and allows complete surface contact during further decontamination procedures. Pre-cleaning should be carried out by trained staff in the CSSD. Machine washing is the preferred option, however some instruments may require washing by hand. Staff performing these procedures must be trained in safe systems of work and wear appropriate protective clothing and gloves. Care should be taken not to produce splashes, high pressure sprays or aerosols.

1. ***High risk:*** Critical items come in close contact with a break in the skin or mucous membrane or introduced into a sterile body area. Items in this category should be sterilized by heat if possible. Heat-labile may be treated

with low-temperature steam and formaldehyde, ethylene oxide, or by irradiation. Liquid chemical sterilant should be used only if other methods are unsuitable.

2. **Intermediate risk:** Semicritical items come in close contact with intact mucous membranes, or body fluids or are contaminated with particularly virulent or readily transmissible microorganisms; or if the items are to be used on highly susceptible patients or sites. In certain circumstances it may be preferable to transfer the items to the "High Risk" category. Disinfection by heat is preferred where this is possible.

3. **Low risk:** Noncritical items in contact with normal and intact skin. Cleaning and drying is usually adequate.

4. **Minimal risk:** Items not in close contact with the patient or their other immediate surroundings. Items in this category are either unlikely to be contaminated with significant numbers of potential pathogens, or transfer to a susceptible site on the patient is unlikely, eg bed-frames, lockers, flower vases, walls, floors, ceilings, sinks and drains. Cleaning and drying is adequate.

CONTROL OF SUBSTANCES HAZARDOUS TO HEALTH (COSHH) REGULATIONS

COSHH is the most recent safety legislation to affect the way in which disinfectants are selected and used in hospitals and health care facilities in the United Kingdom. The COSHH regulations require that the relevant safety precautions are observed when using chemical disinfectants. Therefore, all users of chemical disinfectants must be aware of the correct way to use chemicals to protect themselves from injury. Under the COSHH regulations it is the procedures, rather than substances which should be assessed for risk. The aim of the regulations is to prevent exposure to hazardous substances. For chemical disinfection, the greater risk is from undiluted disinfectants which should be assessed separately from the diluted preparations. Concentrated disinfectants should always be stored and handled with care and appropriate protective clothing and equipment such as gloves, aprons, respiratory and eye protection, etc should be used, where appropriate. Personal protective equipment is required not only to prevent exposure to chemical injury but also to prevent exposure to the microorganisms from cleaning process. For certain chemical disinfectants proper ventilation is required.

Where necessary, the exposure of employees and others who may be exposed should be monitored. The employer has a duty to inform, instruct and train employees and non-employees on the premises in relevant safety matters; this includes the use of chemical disinfectants.

All departments are strongly advised that they should keep the data sheets (available from disinfectant manufacturers) along with other COSHH assessment data. Disinfectants may be harmful, irritant or corrosive and may cause damage by contact with skin, eyes or mucous membranes, by inhalation of vapours or by absorption through the skin. Some may also cause allergic reactions. Environmental disinfectants can damage fabrics, metals and plastics.

Work in an area with easy access to running water and eye-wash bottle. Disinfection should, whenever possible, be carried out in a closed container. Storage containers should never be left open to the atmosphere for longer than absolutely necessary.

Some individuals may be allergic to disinfectants, or more sensitive to them than other people. This may take the form of skin rashes, contact dermatitis or, in rare cases, difficulty in breathing. If you are aware of any disinfectants to which you are sensitive, or suspect that you have reacted to a disinfectant, then you ***must*** inform your line manager who will refer you to the Occupational Health Department for assessment and appropriate action.

Each head of department should ensure that decontamination of all items of equipment in their department are carried out in accordance with the local policy. New items of equipment which are not included in the local manual should have a written protocol which complies both with the manufacturer's recommendations on disinfection and infection control requirements.

Equipment used for sterilization or disinfection ***must*** be commissioned on installation, regularly serviced, maintained and tested in accordance with the manufacturer's instructions and current advice from the Department of Health. A written record must be kept by the head of department. Equipment performance must be maintained to ensure that accepted standards of safety are achieved.

CHEMICAL DISINFECTANTS

There are a number of important factors that must be considered when using chemical disinfectants.

- The efficacy of chemical disinfection is often uncertain and, wherever possible, disinfection by heat is preferable to chemical methods.
- All chemical disinfectants must be clearly labelled and used within the expiry date. They should be freshly prepared. They must be used at the correct concentration and stored in an appropriate container.
- Chemical disinfectant solutions must not be mixed or detergents added unless they are compatible.

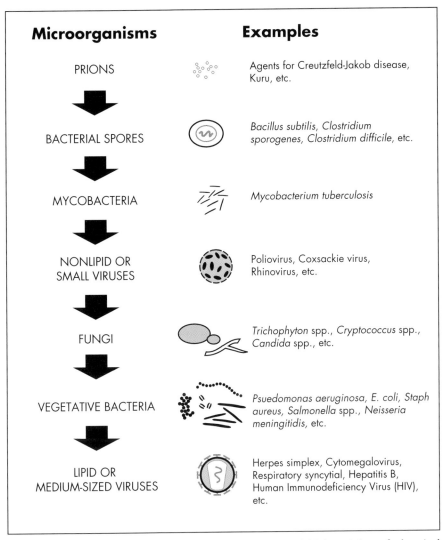

Microorganisms   ## Examples

PRIONS — Agents for Creutzfeld-Jakob disease, Kuru, etc.

BACTERIAL SPORES — Bacillus subtilis, Clostridium sporogenes, Clostridium difficile, etc.

MYCOBACTERIA — Mycobacterium tuberculosis

NONLIPID OR SMALL VIRUSES — Poliovirus, Coxsackie virus, Rhinovirus, etc.

FUNGI — Trichophyton spp., Cryptococcus spp., Candida spp., etc.

VEGETATIVE BACTERIA — Psuedomonas aeruginosa, E. coli, Staph aureus, Salmonella spp., Neisseria meningitidis, etc.

LIPID OR MEDIUM-SIZED VIRUSES — Herpes simplex, Cytomegalovirus, Respiratory syncytial, Hepatitis B, Human Immunodeficiency Virus (HIV), etc.

Figure 3.1 – Descending order of resistance to germicidal activity of chemical disinfectants against various microoganisms.
(Reproduced with modification from Block SS: *Disinfection, Sterilization and Preservation* 4th ed, Philadelphia, Lea & Febiger, 1991).

- Disinfectant or detergent solutions must not be prepared and stored in multi-use containers for occasional use. Solutions prepared and stored in this manner may easily become contaminated with microorganisms; using such solutions will therefore readily contaminate a surface rather than clean it.

- Manufacturer's instructions must be consulted on compatibility of materials with the method of sterilization or disinfection.

DISINFECTANTS AND ANTISEPTICS

Alcohol

Alcohol does not penetrate well into organic matter, especially protein-based, and should therefore be used only on physically clean surfaces.

Uses: Alcohol impregnated wipes are used for disinfection of skin prior to injection. It can be used as a base for other antiseptics, eg chlorhexidine and iodine for pre-operative skin disinfection. Alcohol may be used for disinfecting physically clean equipment or hard surfaces as specified in the local disinfection policy.

Precautions: Alcohol should be stored in a cool place. Alcohol - alcohol mixtures are flammable. Do not allow contact with hot surfaces, flames, electrical equipment or other sources of ignition. If alcohol preparation is used to disinfect pre-operative skin, caution must be exercised whilst using diathermy as it may ignite, causing skin burns if incorrectly used. Therefore all spirit-based skin cleaning and preparation fluids **must** have a cautionary statement, eg *"This preparation contains spirit. When use is to be followed by surgical diathermy do not allow pooling of the fluid to occur and ensure that the skin and surrounding areas are dry"*.

Do not leave bottles uncapped as alcohol vapours irritate mucous membranes, especially in an enclosed space. It may cause eye and skin irritation if used in a large quantity in an enclosed space, therefore its use should be avoided in a poorly ventilated area. If inhaled in large quantities, it may cause headache and drowsiness.

Chlorine-based disinfectants

Hypochlorites are the most widely used of the chlorine disinfectants. They are available in a liquid (sodium hypochlorite), eg "Chloros", "Domestos", "Sterite" and "Milton" or solid (sodium dichloroisocyanurate [NaDCC] or calcium hypochlorite). NaDCC tablets, eg "Presept", "Haz-Tab", "Sanichlor", "Biospot", "Titan" etc are stable and antimicrobial activity of solution prepared from NaDCC tablets may be greater then that of sodium hypochlorite solutions containing the same total available chlorine.

They are fast acting and have broad spectrum of antimicrobial activity. Solutions are unstable at use-dilutions and must therefore be stored according to pharmaceutical recommendations and used **before** the expiry date. They are inactivated by organic matter particularly if used in low concentrations They are incompatible with cationic detergents.

Diluted solutions are unstable and should be freshly prepared daily; decomposition is accelerated by light, heat and heavy metal. Chlorinated disinfectants are corrosive to metal, damaged plastic, rubber and similar components on prolonged contact, or if used at the incorrect dilution. They also bleach fabrics, carpets or soft furnishings.

Uses: It is very active against viruses and is the disinfectant of choice for environmental decontamination following blood spillage from a patient, with known or suspected blood-borne viral infection including hepatitis (B&C), HIV infection. It is incorporated into some non-abrasive cleansing agents which may be used for environmental disinfection on hard surfaces, ie baths or sinks etc. It is used in water treatment and in food preparation areas and milk kitchen. Other uses in hospital and the recommended in-use concentrations are shown in Table 3.3. (See page 62)

Precautions: Chlorinated disinfectants can cause irritation of the skin, eyes and lungs if used frequently in a poorly ventilated area. They should not be used in the presence of formaldehyde as some of the reaction products are carcinogenic. Appropriate protective clothing must be worn when hypochlorite is handled whether in liquid or powdered/granulated form. Skin and eyes should be protected when using undiluted hypochlorite solutions. Store concentrated liquids in pressure-release containers. Sodium hypochlorite should not be mixed with acid or acidic body fluids (eg urine), as toxic chlorine gas will be released.

Phenolics

This group includes "Hycolin", "Stericol" and "Clearsol". These are usually supplied in combination with a detergent to aid the cleaning process. They are not readily inactivated by organic matter, incompatible with cationic detergents and absorbed by rubber and plastics.

Uses: Phenols are used for environmental disinfection. Routine use-dilution for the commonly used clear soluble phenolics ("Hycolin" and "Stericol") is 1% v/v for *"clean"* (low organic soiling) and 2% v/v *"dirty"* (high organic soiling) conditions 2% v/v. It is the agent of choice for mycobacteria including *M.tuberculosis* in the environment. Clear soluble (2%) phenolics are also used in laboratory discard jars in bacteriology.

Precautions: Respiratory irritation may occur if used at concentrations above those listed in the disinfection policy. Appropriate protective clothing must be worn when handling phenolic disinfectants. Skin and eyes must be protected while "making up" or discarding a phenolic solution. Phenolic disinfectants can be absorbed through the skin, therefore skin must be protected during its use. Use latex gloves for intermittent use; medium weight washing up gloves are appropriate for more prolonged contact. Phenol *must not* be used on equipment that may come in contact with skin or mucous membranes. It *must not* be used in the Special Care Baby Unit to disinfect incubators and other items because of the risk of occurrence of hyperbilirubinemia in infants. It may taint food therefore *do not* use on food preparation surfaces.

Aldehydes

Glutaraldehyde

Most preparations of glutaraldehyde are non-corrosive to metals and other materials and inactivation by organic matter is very low. Alkaline solutions require activation; once activated they remain active for 2-4 weeks depending on the brand or preparation used and the frequency of use. Acidic solutions are stable and do not require activation, but slower in activity than alkaline buffered solutions.

Uses: 2% glutaraldehyde ("Cidex", "Asep") is used to disinfect heat-sensitive items, ie endoscopes.

Precautions: Glutaraldehyde is an eye and nasal irritant and may cause respiratory illness (asthma) and allergic dermatitis. Glutaraldehyde should not be used in an area with little or no ventilation as exposure is likely to be at or above the current Occupational Exposure Standards (OES: 0.2 ppm/0.7 mgm^{-3}, 10 minutes only). Eye protection, a plastic apron and gloves must be worn when glutaraldehyde liquid is made up, disposed of, or when immersing instruments. Latex gloves may be worn and discarded after use if the duration of contact with glutaraldehyde is brief, ie less than 5 minutes. For longer duration, nitrile gloves must be worn. It should be stored away from heat sources and in containers with close-fitting lids.

Formaldehyde

Uses: Formaldehyde is used mainly as a gaseous fumigant to disinfect safety cabinets in the laboratory and to fumigate rooms of patients with highly dangerous and transmissible infectious disease who are kept in strict isolation. These uses may only be carried out by persons fully trained and competent in the correct procedure. Arrangements for this process may only be made with prior consultation with the Infection Control Doctor.

Precautions: Formaldehyde is a potent eye and nasal irritant and may cause respiratory distress and allergic dermatitis. Gloves, goggles and aprons should be worn when preparing and disposing of formaldehyde solutions. When formalin is used regularly for disinfection, advice from the Control of Substances Hazardous to Health (COSHH) Team should be obtained as monitoring may be required.

Peracetic acid

A special advantage of peracetic acid is its harmless decomposition products and lack of residue. It remains effective in the presence of organic matter and is sporacidal even at low temperatures. Peracetic acid can corrode copper, brass, bronze, plain steel and galvanised iron, but these effects can be reduced by additives and pH modification. It is considered unstable particularly when diluted. An automated machine using peracetic acid chemically sterilises medical, surgical (eg endoscopes, arthroscopes) and dental instruments. It is more effective than glutaraldehyde at penetrating organic matter, eg biofilms. It is known to be highly corrosive and its use as a disinfectant in its natural state is therefore limited unless there is a corrosion inhibitor in the formulation. "Nu-Cidex" is stabilised peracetic acid solution with corrosion inhibitor. It is used as a cold sterilant/disinfectant solution to disinfect endoscopes. The solution is activated to provide the appropriate in-use strength. Once prepared the current manufacturer's recommendation is that it should be used within 24 hours.

Hydrogen peroxide

Hydrogen peroxide and peroxygen compounds, "Virkon", have low toxicity and irritancy. Hydrogen peroxide has been used in concentration from 3-6% for the disinfection of contact lenses, tonometer biprisms, etc. Hydrogen peroxide has not been widely used for endoscope disinfection because of concerns that its oxidising properties may be harmful to some components of the endoscope. Peroxygen compounds, where of low irritancy, are sometimes used for disinfecting small spills and for laboratory equipment where other methods are impractical. Manufacturer's approval should be obtained before using on equipment where corrosion may present problems, eg endoscopes, centrifuges etc.

Chlorhexidine

This group includes "Hibiscrub", "Hibitane" etc. Chlorhexidine is inactivated by soap, organic matter and anionic detergents. It also stains fabrics brown in the presence of chlorine-based disinfectants.

Uses: Used exclusively as an antiseptic which involves contact with skin and mucous membranes. Chlorhexidine solutions are usually combined with detergent which is used for hand disinfection or with alcohol ("Hibisol") which is useful if rapid disinfection is required for physically clean hands. It is combined with alcohol for pre-operative skin disinfection and with cetramide ("Savalon") for cleaning dirty wounds.

Precautions: Chlorhexidine is relatively non-toxic. It **must not** be allowed to come in contact with the brain, meninges, eye or middle ear.

Iodine and Iodophors

This group includes aqueous iodine, tincture of iodine, "Betadine", "Disadine" "Videne", "Phoraid", etc. It is inactivated by organic matter and may corrode metals.Iodophors do not stain skin and are non-irritant.

Uses: Alcoholic preparations containing iodine and iodophors are suitable for pre-operative skin preparation. Povidone iodine detergent preparations are for surgical hand-disinfection.

Precautions: Use gloves for prolonged handling of iodine/iodophors preparation. An alcoholic iodophor is less irritant than an alcohol/iodine mixture. Tincture of iodine and aqueous iodine solutions can cause skin reactions in some individuals, therefore iodophors solution is usually preferred.

Quaternary Ammonium Compounds

All Quaternary Ammonium Compounds (QACs) have detergent properties. They are inactivated by soaps, anionic detergents and organic matter.

Uses: QACs (with or without chlorhexidine solutions) may be used for cleaning dirty wounds. QACs are *not* recommended as an environmental disinfectant.

Precautions: QACs inhibit the growth of bacteria (bacteriostatic) but do not kill them. Contamination and growth of Gram-negative bacilli in dilute solutions is, therefore, a problem which can be avoided by using single-use sachets where practical. Discard any unused solutions immediately after use and do not prepare in use dilutions in the clinical area. Obtain the correct strength from your pharmacy. Decanting from one container and topping-up should be avoided. This can result in contamination with airborne contaminants and growth of Gram-negative bacteria which may then colonize the wound. Liquid should be stored in closed bottles until immediately before use. Water-baths should be disinfected after use.

Hexachlorophane

Hexachlorophane is a chlorinated bisphenol. Hexachlorophane is not fast acting and its rate of killing is classified as slow to intermediate. The major advantage of hexachlorophane is its persistence. Soaps and other organic materials have little effect. Hexachlorophane [(0.33%) "Ster-Zac"] powder is used to protect colonization with *Staph.aureus* in neonates without significant toxicity risk. It has good residual effect on the skin and can be used by adults for surgical hand disinfection or during staphylococcal outbreak. Use of hexachlorophane on broken skin or mucous membranes or for routine total body bathing is contraindicated.

Triclosan

Triclosan ("Manusept", "Aquasept") phenol or Irgasan is a diphenyl ether. It can be absorbed through intact skin but appears to be non-allergenic and non-mutagenic with short term use. Its speed of killing is intermediate but has excellent persistent activity on skin. Its activity is only minimally affected by organic matter. It is commonly used in deodorant soaps and health care hand washes. It has a similar range of antimicrobial activity as Hexachlorophane but exhibits no documented toxicity in neonates.

Table 3.1 – Antimicrobial activity and summary of properties of disinfectants.

Disinfectant	Antimicrobial activity					Other properties			
	Bacteria	Mycobacteria	Spores	Viruses		Stability	Inactivation by organic matter	Corrosive/ damaging	Irritant/ Sensitizing
				Enveloped	Non Enveloped				
Alcohol 60-70% (ethanol or isopropanol)	+++	+++	-	++	++	Yes (in closed container)	Yes (fixative)	Slight (lens cements)	No
Chlorine releasing agents 0.5-1% available chlorine	+++	+++	+++	+++	+++	No (<1 day)	Yes	Yes	Yes
Clear soluble phenolics 1-2%	+++	++	-	++	+	Yes	No	Slight	Yes
Glutaraldehyde 2%	+++	+++	+++	+++	+++	Moderately (14-28 days)	No (fixative)	No	Yes
Peracetic acid 0.2-0.35%	+++	+++	+++	+++	+++	No (<1 day)	No	Slight	Slight
Peroxygen compounds* 3-6%	+++	±	±	+++	±	Moderately (7 days)	Yes	Slight	No

Good = +++, Moderate = ++, Poor = +, Variable ±, None = -

*activity varies with concentration

Table 3.2 – Antimicrobial activity of antiseptics.

Antiseptics	Bacteria	Mycobacteria	Fungi	Virus
Alcohols	+++	+++	+++	+++
Chlorhexidine 4% aqueous	+++	++	++	+++
Hexachlorophane 3% aqueous	+++	+	+	+
Iodine compounds and Iodophors	+++	++	+++	+++
Triclosan	+++	++	+	++
Quaternary ammonia compounds	++	±	-	+

Good = +++, Moderate = ++, Poor = +, Variable = ±, None = -

Table 3.3 – Uses of hypochlorite and strengths of solution.

Uses	Dilution of stock solution*	Available %	chlorine ppm
	Undiluted	10	100,000
Blood spills	1 in 10	1.0	10,000
Laboratory discard jars	1 in 40	0.25	2,500
General environmental disinfection	1 in 100	0.1	1,000
Disinfection of clean instruments	1 in 200	0.05	500
Infant feeding utensils, catering surfaces and equipment	1 in 800	0.0125	125

Note: * Approximate values of some undiluted brands, ie "Chloros", "Domestos", "Sterite" etc, are Sodium hypochlorite 10% w/v (100,000 ppm av Cl_2) and undiluted "Milton" is Sodium hypochlorite 1% w/v (10,000 ppm av Cl_2)

Reproduced with permission from Ayliffe GAJ et al. Chemical Disinfection in Hospitals, 2 ed, PHLS,1993.

DISINFECTION OF FLEXIBLE FIBREOPTIC ENDOSCOPES

The number of endoscopic procedures used on patients for diagnostic and therapeutic reasons is increasing each year, resulting in, increasing problems with infections. Although the overall incidence of infection following endoscopy is very low, it can only be avoided by maintaining the highest standards while decontaminating endoscopes after each use. Endoscopes can be categorised by their design into two types:

1. *Rigid endoscopes* are bronchoscope and arthroscopes which are relatively easy to clean, disinfect and sterilize. Sterilization is the preferred process for rigid endoscopes but many are not heat tolerant, therefore as an alternative, rigid endoscopes may be disinfected using liquid chemicals or low temperature steam.

2. *Flexible endoscopes* are bronchoscope and gastrointestinal endoscopes. They are more complex and, therefore, are difficult to clean, disinfect and sterilize. Flexible endoscopes are heat sensitive and are damaged when exposed to temperatures in excess of 60°C, a temperature well below that considered suitable for thermal disinfection. Therefore, chemical disinfection or sterilization must be performed at low temperature.

Table 3.5 – Summary of disinfection of endoscopes.

Endoscope	Contact time in 2% activated alkaline glutaraldehyde
Flexible Bronchoscopes (British Thoracic Society)	20 minutes between patients, beginning and end of list. 60 minutes on known or suspected case of pulmonary. tuberculosis or before immunocompromised patient.
Cystoscopes (British Association of Urological Surgeons)	10 minutes (at least) between patients, beginning and end of list. 60 minutes on known or suspected mycobacterial infection.
Gastrointestinal endoscope (British Socitey of Gastroenterology) *Under revision.*	4 minutes between patients. 20 minutes at beginning and end of list. 60 minutes after if used on AIDS/immunocompromised patient.
Artroscopes, laparoscopes (Hospital Infection Research Laboratory)	10 minutes (at least) between patients.

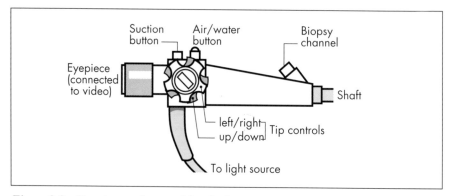

Figure 3.2 – Eyepiece and control head of gastrointestinal fiberoptic endoscope. (Reproduced with permission from Cotton PB, Williams CB: *Practical gastrointestinal endoscopy* 3rd ed. Boston: Blackwell, 1990)

Decontamination

The cleaning, disinfection and sterilization of all endoscopes must be carried out by fully trained staff according to the written protocol based on the manufacturer's recommendations. It is recommended that staff handling used endoscopes or working in the endoscopy unit should be immunized against Hepatitis B infection. Effective decontamination of endoscopes requires input from:

- Clinician or the user of the instrument who is familiar with the risks associated with the procedure.

- Infection Control personnel who are responsible for advising on the selection and use of a suitable decontamination process.

- Endoscopy nurse, sterile services personnel or other person responsible for processing.

- Instrument manufacturer or supplier who is familiar with the design and function of the item and its compatibility with heat and chemicals.

Cleaning: Thorough manual cleaning of the instrument and its internal channels with detergent is the most important part of the disinfection procedure. Without this dry residual organic material, such as blood or mucous, may prevent penetration of the disinfectant. It also ensures better contact between the disinfectant or sterilant and, removal of any remaining microorganisms in subsequent stages of decontamination. Cleaning with warm water and a neutral or enzymatic detergent is recommended, though advice on suitable cleaning agents should be sought from the endoscope's manufacturer. The detergent should be changed at a frequency to prevent its contamination with organic matter. It is important that the instrument is in full working order and that a "Leak Test" has been performed to ensure that it is watertight prior to any cleaning procedure.

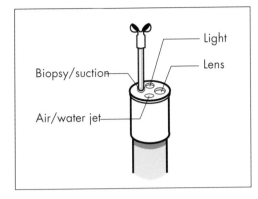

Biopsy/suction

Air/water jet

Light

Lens

Figure 3.3 – Part of the deflectable tip of gastrointestinal fiberoptic endoscope.
(Reproduced with permission from Cotton PB, Williams CB: *Practical gastrointestinal endoscopy* 3rd ed. Boston: Blackwell, 1990).

There are many machines available that are capable of cleaning as well as disinfecting endoscopes. However, it is essential that initial manual cleaning, at the point of use, is performed to ensure the effectiveness of subsequent processing and prevent the machine and the disinfectant becoming contaminated with excess organic matter or body fluids. Appropriate cleaning brushes dedicated for the purpose should be used for all accessible channels and ports. Staff with specialised training and knowledge of the instrument are essential for this to be done effectively.

Ultrasonic washers may be used for most rigid endoscope components and accessories with the exception of the telescope. All lumens should be irrigated, after ultrasonic cleansing to remove dislodged organic matter. Irrigation pumps are available for flushing instrument lumens and components.

Cleaning and disinfection or sterilization should be undertaken before the endoscopy list, between each patient, at the end of the list and prior to inspection, service or repair. A record should be maintained of the cleaning, disinfection and sterilization process for each endoscope.

Disinfection: Endoscopes which are passed into normally sterile body cavities must be sterilized prior to use. Endoscopes which come into contact with intact mucous membranes but do not invade sterile cavities can be decontaminated using high-level disinfection by the head of the department.

Immersion in a suitable liquid chemical disinfectant is the most widely used procedure for the decontamination of flexible and heat sensitive rigid endoscopes. The most widely used agents are 2% activated glutaraldehyde. Glutaraldehydes are irritants, therefore nitrile gloves and a plastic apron must be worn; eye protection is necessary if splashing is likely, eg when filling and emptying immersion tanks (See page 58).

The problems associated with the use of the most commonly used disinfectant, glutaraldehyde, have prompted the development of non-aldehyde alternatives. Examples of such are those based on peracetic acid, although, unfortunately, these may be more damaging to some instrument components than glutaraldehyde. It is essential that advice is sought from the endoscope manufacturer on compatibility with any new disinfectant or process. The decision as to which disinfectant to use for a particular situation is ultimately made at a local level.

There is some discrepancy between the various professional recommendations with respect to the disinfectant contact time (Table 3.4 page 63). Furthermore, at these contact times may be a variance with the recommendations of the manufacturer of the chosen disinfectant.

Problems due to inadequate decontamination

Major problems leading to inadequate decontamination are:

1. *Inadequate cleaning:* Failure to remove deposits of blood, faeces, tissue, mucous, microorganisms, film or slime may result in infection, misdiagnosis or instrument malfunction.

2. *Automatic washer/disinfector systems:* A number of factors have been associated with contamination of machines:
   - inadequate cleaning and maintenance of the machine.
   - the use of static water, ie within pipework or tank.
   - the use of a water supply of poor microbiological quality.
   - the use of hard water.
   - inadequate pre-cleaning of the endoscope.
   - the formation of biofilm within the machine.

   All tank and fluid pathways in endoscope washer/disinfectors should be regularly drained, cleaned and disinfected to prevent colonization of the fluid pathway which could be responsible for misdiagnosis of a patient's infection. Seek advice from the manufacturer of the washer/disinfector on compatible cleaning agents and disinfectants to ensure no damage to the machine occurs. Disinfection should be performed at the start of each session prior to using the endoscope washer/disinfector. Water used to rinse endoscopes following disinfection must be of a suitable quality with respect to hardness and freedom from microbiological contamination. It should preferably be filtered through a bacteria-retaining filter so that the instrument does not become recontaminated.

   A record must be kept of the number of washing cycles to ensure that the disinfectant is not unreasonably diluted or neutralized by organic matter. Appropriate records on disinfection of the equipment must be maintained by the department.

3. *Microbiological quality of water or other fluids:* Hardness of water resulting in the build up of lime scale on the internal pipework of the washer/disinfector and poor microbiological quality result in microbial contamination. The use of pre-sterilized bottled water for stand alone machines and the use of pre-treated water for mains connected machines. Tap water may contain microbes including *Pseudomonas* and *Mycobacterium* spp and there are many reports of procedure acquired infection with these organisms via contaminated rinse water. Mis-diagnosis of tuberculosis has been reported due to contamination of the instruments with environmental mycobacteria from the rinse water which subsequently contaminated bronchial washing sent for culture. Therefore, sterile water is recommended for the final rinsing of all types of endoscope to be used for all invasive procedures.

4. *Renewal of disinfectant:* Serial processing of endoscopes in automated systems may reduce disinfectant potency due to constant dilution of the disinfectant by wet instruments. Therefore, disinfectant should be changed frequently; at least weekly or sooner, depending on usage and its contamination with organic matter. The concentration of glutaraldehyde in the solution should not be allowed to fall below 1.5% and solutions must not be used beyond the manufacturer's recommended post-activation life. Test kits are available which indicate glutaraldehyde concentration. The rinse water should also be changed regularly to avoid build-up of glutaraldehyde on the instrument and eyepiece assembly, as residues may cause skin and eye irritation.

After decontamination, final rinsing of endoscopes and accessories with sterile water is important as many of the agents used for this process deposit toxic residues which must be adequately rinsed off before the endoscope can be used.

DECONTAMINATION OF SUCTION EQUIPMENT

Suction systems can either be **Fixed** unit which can be used with a re-usable (suction jar) or disposable (liner) reservoir or **Portable** unit which is normally used with re-usable (suction jar) reservoir, but may be adapted for use with a disposable (liner) reservoir. Suction tubing, handles and catheters are all disposable.

Suction containers or reservoir can either be disposable or non-disposable. When emptying non-disposable (suction jar) reservoir the following precautions should be taken:

- A plastic apron and household gloves should be worn for emptying the suction jar. In addition, eye protection must be worn if the patient belongs to *high risk* group. A high filtration mask must be worn for a patient with pulmonary tuberculosis.

- The jar must be disconnected from the vacuum system, carried carefully to the dirty utility room and poured gently into the sluice hopper. The contents should be flushed with copious amounts of running water.

- The jar should be rinsed, and then washed with a neutral pH detergent and hot water solution. It must be rinsed again in fresh water and dried with disposable wipes.

- A weak solution of sodium bicarbonate (mucolytic agent) may be used to help remove mucous material. Alternatively the suction jar may be machine washed in a washer/disinfector unit.

- The bottle should be emptied when full and cleaned at least daily irrespective of the amount of fluid aspirate. Fresh tubing should be attached just prior to use.

When handling disposable (liner) reservoir the following precautions should be taken:

- A plastic apron and gloves should be worn.

- The suction reservoir should be disconnected from the vacuum system and sealed correctly according to manufacturer's instruction.

- The liner must be placed upright in an appropriate container, sealed securely and transported as clinical waste.

- The disposal container must clearly indicate the contents to ensure care is taken during transport to prevent damage or spillage of contents. In addition the container must be clearly marked with the hospital and ward or department.

Practical Points

- The routine use of a disinfectant is unnecessary for cleaning suction jars. The organic matter in the contents readily inactivate disinfectants, therefore addition of disinfectants will only lengthen the process and it will be of no advantage. The only exception to this is when the patient has pulmonary tuberculosis or other infectious diseases. In such cases it is preferable to send the equipment to the CSSD for disinfection.

- A fresh single-use disposable suction catheter must be used each time a patient undergoes tracheo-bronchial aspiration. Yankaeur suction catheters or handles can be re-used on the same patient provided they are flushed after use by drawing a sodium bicarbonate solution through the tip followed by aspirating the air for 20 seconds, drying with a disposable tissue and storing in a protective cover.

- Approximately 10ml of an anti-foaming agent (eg "Foamtrol" or "Medeform") may be added just prior to use to prevent excessive foaming of the bottle contents, which may wet the filter and enter the pump mechanism.

- The filter should be changed between patients or if it becomes moist or discoloured or used by an infected patient, eg HIV/AIDS, blood-borne hepatitis (B&C), tuberculosis, etc. If in doubt seek advice from the Infection Control Nurse.

- When the suction unit is not in use, the bottle should be kept dry and the catheter should not be connected until it is required. The machine should be covered with a dust proof cover if not in use. Suction machines must be serviced according to the manufacturer's instructions and records retained by the head of the department.

DECONTAMINATION OF EQUIPMENT PRIOR TO INSPECTION, SERVICE OR REPAIR

Equipment and items which have been contaminated by contact with blood and high risk body fluids, pathological specimens, or exposure to patients in isolation will require decontamination prior to examination by third parties who perform inspection, service or repair.

Heads of department are responsible for the provision and implementation of policy to prevent transmission of infection from contact with contaminated equipment and are also responsible to protect anyone handling equipment which may have become contaminated with corrosive, irritant, toxic, cytotoxic or radio active agents as well.

All decontamination procedures should be undertaken by suitably qualified, trained, and supervised staff using suitable equipment. The method of decontamination to be used must be one that does not damage the article or any of its components and could include steam sterilization, dry heat, or chemical methods. In cases of doubt about the appropriate method, advice should be sought from:

- the manufacturer or agent.
- hospital engineering staff.
- the sterile services manager (CSSD).
- a member of the Infection Control Team.

A record of the procedures or safety precautions used should be kept in the equipment log book. A written declaration of decontamination status must be provided. If the equipment is to leave the premises, the certificate/statement should be enclosed in an envelope affixed to the outside of the package.

In certain situations equipment may not be decontaminated before inspection, service or repair, either because the equipment is subject to investigation as the result of a complaint or it may not be adequately decontaminated without engineering assistance. In such cases, the advice of the investigating body or engineering department should be sought. If such an item is to leave the premises the following precautions must be taken:

- a prior warning should be given to the intended recipient.
- the condition of the item should be clearly labelled on the outer packaging.
- the packaging should be suitably robust to ensure that the inner pack cannot contaminate the outer pack or become damaged in transport.
- the agreement of any transporter may be required.

DECONTAMINATION OF INFECTIOUS SPILLS

Spills of blood and high risk body fluids should be removed as soon as possible and the area washed with detergent and dried. Single-use disposable gloves and a plastic apron must be worn for dealing with infectious spills. Glass fragments **must** be picked up with forceps or use disposable (or autoclavable) scoop or dustpan and brush; eye protection should be worn. A spillage from a patient with a known or suspected blood borne viral infection, eg Hepatitis (B&C) or HIV infection should be disinfected using a chlorine-based disinfectant, ie hypochlorite or NaDCC granules.

Splashes and drips

Splashes and small drips of blood should be wiped up using a paper towel soaked in hypochlorite (10,000 ppm a Cl_2) solution.

Procedure

1. Wear non-sterile gloves for this procedure.
2. The gloves and paper towels should be discarded into a yellow plastic bag as clinical waste for incineration.
3. Hands should be washed and dried immediately after removing gloves.
4. Treated surface should be rinsed with clean water (since hypochlorite solution is corrosive).
5. Drie the surface with disposable paper towels.

Larger spills

Procedure

1. Larger spills should be sprinkled with sodium dichloroisocyanurate (NaDCC) granules until the fluid is absorbed if the quantity is $\leq$ 30ml. For spills >30ml, cover the spillage with paper towels to absorb all liquid and carefully pour a freshly prepared hypochlorite (10,000 ppm av Cl_2) solution.

2. Leave the spill for a contact period of 2-5 minutes to allow for disinfection.

3. Depending on the method used, either scoop up the absorbed granules or lift the soiled paper towels and discard into a yellow plastic bag as clinical waste for incineration.

4. Wipe the surface area with fresh hypochlorite (10,000 ppm av Cl_2) solution and rinse with clean water.

5. Dry the surface with disposable paper towels.

6. Remove gloves and plastic apron and discard as clinical waste for incineration.

7. Wash hands and dry immediately.

TERMINAL CLEANING OF ROOM

Terminal cleaning of a room is indicated when a patient has been under source isolation and is discharged or transferred to another area. The following procedure should be followed:

1. Domestic staff must wear a disposable plastic apron and appropriate colour coded household type gloves.

2. Terminal cleaning should commence only after the patient and his/her possessions have been removed from the room or the area.

3. Discard any disposable items or equipment as appropriate.

4. Seal yellow clinical waste bags before leaving the room and discard as clinical waste for incineration.

5. Place all linen (including bed linen, curtains, screen, soft furnishings etc) into the appropriate bags and treat as "Infected Linen". Bags must be sealed before leaving the room or the area.

6. Remove any items of nursing equipment to the dirty utility area for cleaning and disinfection. All autoclavable items should be sent to CSSD.

7. The bed mattresses should be wiped with warm water and detergent and

dried thoroughly. If disinfectant is indicated, wipe with freshly prepared hypochlorite (1000 ppm av Cl$_2$) solution.

8. Dust the high ledges, window frames and curtain tracks.

9. Vacuum clean fixtures, fittings and floor. Only a suitable vacuum cleaner with a high filter mechanism must be used.

10. Wet clean all ledges, fixtures and fittings, including taps and door handles.

11. Wash sink with hypochlorite/detergent cleanser, rinse and dry thoroughly.

12. Wash floor and spot clean walls with detergent solution. Rinse and dry thoroughly.

13. Open windows, if required, to facilitate thorough drying of all surfaces.

14. The room may be used again for other patients when all surfaces are clean and dry.

If the patient is isolated in an open ward near a sink, then the entire surrounding area up to the next bed, including curtains, should be cleaned as above. Seek advice from the Infection Control Nurse.

Table 3.5 – Disinfection procedures for individual items and equipment.

Equipment or site	Routine or preferred method	Acceptable alternative or additional recommendations
Airways and endotracheal tubes	Single-use disposable or heat sterilize in the CSSD.	Use single-use disposable item or heat sterilize for patients with known infection, eg tuberculosis, AIDS, etc.
Ampoules	Wipe neck with a 70% isopropyl alcohol impregnated swab and allow to dry before opening or piercing.	When a sterile ampoule exterior is required, it will be processed by the CSSD, by agreement with medical and pharmaceutical staff. Do not immerse an ampoule in a disinfectant solution.
Babies feeding bottles and teats	Use pre-sterilized or terminally heat-treated feeds. *Non-disposable bottles*: wash thoroughly, rinse and place in fresh hypochlorite (125 ppm av Cl_2) solution for 30 minutes.	Chemical disinfectant should be used only when other methods are unavailable. Non-disposable bottles which originate from a milk kitchen must be returned there for disinfection.
Baths	*Non-infected patients*: Clean with detergent or use a non-abrasive cream cleanser to remove stain or scum if necessary. Rinse and dry after cleaning, before and after use.	*Infected patients*: Disinfect by cleaning with a chlorine-based agent or a non-abrasive chlorine releasing powder. *Patients with open wounds*: For patients with unhealed wounds and those who are immunocompromised, disinfect before use with a non-abrasive hypochlorite powder. Apply powder to a wet surface, rinse thoroughly and dry.
Bath water	Do not add an antiseptic bath additive routinely.	For staphylococcal dispersers seek advice from a member of the Infection Control Team.
Beds and cots	Wash with detergent and dry.	*Infected patients*: Use hypochlorite (1,000 ppm av Cl_2) solution for disinfection. Do not use phenolic disinfectants on infant cots, prams or incubators as residual fumes may cause respiratory irritation.

Table 3.5 – Continued

Equipment or site	Routine or preferred method	Acceptable alternative or additional recommendations
Bedframes	Wash with detergent and dry.	Infected patients: Wipe with disinfectant, wash with detergent, rinse and dry.
Bedpans and urinals	Heat disinfect in a washer-disinfector, (80°C for 1 min). After removal from the machine ensure that there is no visible soiling. Clean if necessary and store dry.	Infected patients: Gloves and plastic aprons must be worn when handling contaminated items from infected patients. Alternatively, single-use disposable items may be used. These should always be disposed of into a macerator unit.
Bowls (washing)	Individual wash bowls should be available for each patient. After each use, wash with detergent, rinse, dry and store inverted and tilted forward to avoid trapping of water which may harbour microorganisms.	Infected patients: After thorough cleaning, disinfect by wiping with a disinfectant solution.
Bowls (surgical, sterile)	Return to CSSD for autoclaving.	
Bowls (vomit)	Empty and rinse. Wash with detergent and hot water, rinse and dry.	For infected patient [see above under Bowls (washing)].
Breast pumps	For individual patient's use only. Wash with detergent and water then rinse. Immerse in hypochlorite (125 ppm av Cl_2) solution for 30 minutes. Autoclave before use by other patients.	For communal use, return to CSSD for autoclaving after each patient's use.
Carpets	Suction clean daily with a vacuum cleaner with an effective filter. Shampoo periodically by hot water extraction or when soiled.	For known contaminated spills, disinfect with an agent that does not damage carpet and then clean with a detergent. Seek advice from the Infection Control Nurse.

Table 3.5 – Continued

Equipment or site	Routine or preferred method	Acceptable alternative or additional recommendations
Cheatle forceps	Do not use.	If used in an exceptional circumstance, autoclave daily and store in a fresh 1% clear soluble phenolic disinfectant which must be changed daily.
Cleaning equipment	*Mops*: the detachable heads of used mops must be machine laundered, thermally disinfected and dried daily. *Mop bucket*: wash with detergent. Rinse, dry and store inverted. *Scrubbing machine*: drain reservoir after use and store dry.	Colour coded cleaning equipment should be used for each area, ie clinical, non-clinical, kitchen and sanitary area according to the local policy.
Commodes	Wash seat daily with detergent and hot water and dry with a disposable paper towel. After each use the seat of the commode should be cleaned with a large alcohol impregnated wipe.	If faecal contamination has occurred, remove soil with tissue. Wash with detergent and hot water. Wipe with disinfectant, wash, rinse and dry.
Crockery and cutlery	Machine wash with rinse temperature above 80°C and dry or hand wash in detergent and hot water (approx. 60°C), rinse and allow to dry thoroughly. Rubber gloves will be required at this temperature.	*Infected patients*: For patients with enteric infections or open pulmonary tuberculosis, heat disinfect in a dishwasher.
Drains	Clean regularly as outlined in the maintenance programme. Chemical disinfection is not required.	When blockage occurs, contact environmental Works and Maintenance Department.
Duvets	Launder to thermal disinfection temperatures.	Launder after each patient use, weekly or if visible soiled.

Table 3.5 – *Continued*

Equipment or site	Routine or preferred method	Acceptable alternative or additional recommendations
Endoscopes	*Flexible fibreoptic endoscopes:* See page 63.	
	Arthroscopes & Laparoscopes: Clean and wash thoroughly. Rinse, dry and send to CSSD for sterilization.	
	If this is not possible, a 10 minutes exposure to 2% alkaline glutaraldehyde is used. The instrument must be dismantled and thoroughly cleaned before disinfection and rinsed in sterile water afterwards.	If used on a patient where tuberculosis is suspected, then the contact time with 2% alkaline glutaraldehyde must be extended to 60 minutes.
	Procto/Sigmoidoscope: Clean and wash thoroughly. Rinse and dry and send it to CSSD for sterilization or use disposable, if available.	
	If this is not possible, a 10 minutes exposure to 2% alkaline glutaraldehyde is used. The instrument must be dismantled and thoroughly cleaned before disinfection and rinsed in sterile water afterwards.	If used on a patient where tuberculosis is suspected, then the contact time with 2% alkaline glutaraldehyde must be extended to 60 minutes.
Enteral feeding lines	Single-use disposable.	
Floors (dry cleaning)	Vacuum clean or use a dust-attracting dry mop.	Never use brooms in patient areas.
Floors (wet cleaning)	Wash with a detergent solution Disinfection is not routinely required.	If contaminated, disinfect and clean as outlined on page 70.
Fixtures & fittings	In clinical areas damp dust daily with detergent solution.	In known contaminated and special areas, damp dust with a disinfectant solution.
Furniture & ledges	In clinical areas damp dust daily with warm water and detergent.	

Table 3.5 – Continued

Equipment or site	Routine or preferred method	Acceptable alternative or additional recommendations
Humidifiers	Clean and sterilize device between patients and fill with sterile water which must be changed every 24 hours or sooner if necessary. Single-use disposables are available.	Seek advice from the Infection Control Team.
Infant incubators	After use, wash all removable parts and thoroughly clean with detergent. Rinse and dry thoroughly using disposable paper towels.	*Infected patients:* After cleaning, wipe with 70% isopropyl alcohol impregnated wipe or with hypochlorite (125 ppm av Cl_2) solution. Aerate the incubator before re-use. *Do not* use phenolic disinfectant. Alcohol may damage the plastic surfaces. Please refer to the manufacturer's instructions.
Instruments (surgical, sterile)	Return to CSSD for machine washing and sterilization. Transport safely in a closed rigid container.	Contaminated instruments should be cleaned by trained staff in CSSD before sterilization.
Laryngoscope blade	Wash with detergent, rinse, dry and wipe with an alcohol impregnated wipe.	Contaminated instruments should be sterilized in CSSD.
Linen	Refer to the local policy.	
Locker tops	Treat as "Fixtures and Fittings"	
Mattresses & pillows	Wash water impermeable cover with hot water and detergent solution, rinse and dry.	Should be protected by a waterproof cover. *Infected patients:* Disinfect with a disinfectant solution. Allow two minutes contact time then rinse and dry. Do not disinfect unnecessarily as this damages mattress cover.

Table 3.5 – Continued

Equipment or site	Routine or preferred method	Acceptable alternative or additional recommendations
Mops (dish)	Do not use.	
Mops (dry, dust attracting)	Do not use if overloaded or for more than 1-2 days without reprocessing or washing. Alternatively a single-use disposable cover may be used and disposed of after each use.	Non-disposable dust mop covers must be vacuumed after each use. Single-use covers should be of the type which is impregnated with mineral oil to enhance dust attracting properties
Mops (wet)	Mop heads must be changed daily. Reprocess by machine washing to thermal disinfection temperature and tumble dry.	If chemical disinfection is required, rinse in water, immerse in hypochlorite (1,000 ppm av Cl_2) solution for at least 30 minutes.
Nail brushes	Use only if essential. Heat disinfect in CSSD after each use or use sterile pre-packed single-use disposable.	Do not soak in a disinfectant solution. Never use a nail brush to scrub skin.
Nebulizers	Change and reprocess device between patients by using sterilization or a high level of disinfection or use single-use disposable items. Fill with sterile water only.	
Oxygen tents	Wash with hot water detergent solution, rinse well and dry thoroughly.	Store covered with clean plastic sheeting in a clean area.
Pillows	Use only with water impermeable cover. Treat as "mattresses".	Damaged pillows must be replaced immediately.
Razors (electric)	Detach head, clean thoroughly, and immerse in 70% isopropyl alcohol for 10 minutes, remove and allow to dry between each patient.	Ideally each patient should have their own shaving equipment or use single-use disposable.
Razors (safety and open)	Use disposable or autoclave with single-use disposable head.	For clinical shaving, use clipper.
Rhino/ laryngoscope	Clean the blade thoroughly with detergent and hot water. Dry thoroughly and wipe with a 70% alcohol impregnated wipe.	In cases of suspected/confirmed transmissible infection or visible . blood, the blade should be sterilised before further use.

Table 3.5 – *Continued*

Equipment or site	Routine or preferred method	Acceptable alternative or additional recommendations
Rooms (terminal cleaning)	Wash surfaces with detergent solution.	*Transmissible Infection:* disinfect surface with disinfectant solution, wash with detergent, rinse and dry. See page 71.
Scissors	If not required sterile, wipe before and after use with a 70% alcohol impregnated wipe.	
Shaving brushes	Do not use for clinical shaving.	Use brushless cream or shaving foam. Patients may use their own brush for face shaves, it should be rinsed under running water and stored dry.
Sheepskins	*Synthetic:* return to laundry department for washing in the usual way. *Natural fibre:* for individual use only.	Seek advice from the Infection Control Nurse.
Soap	*Bar Soap:* store dry in a soap drainer. *Liquid Soap:* should be supplied in a dispensing container. Avoid "topping up".	See page 161.
Sputum containers	Use disposable only. Seal and discard as clinical waste daily or sooner if required.	
Suction equipment	Following use, the reservoir should be emptied into the sluice hopper, washed with hot water and detergent, rinsed and store dried. Wear a plastic apron and non-sterile disposable gloves for this procedure. The reservoir of the suction apparatus should be kept empty and dry when not in use.	When using a disposable system, great care is required to ensure the safe disposal of liners according to waste disposal policy. For infected patients seek advice from the Infection Control Nurse. Refer to page 67.

Table 3.5 – Continued

Equipment or site	Routine or preferred method	Acceptable alternative or additional recommendations
Thermometers (electronic)	Use a single-use sleeve and change after each use.	Do not use without sleeve, or on patients with an infectious disease.
Thermometers (oral)	*Individual thermometers:* wipe with a 70% isopropyl alcohol impregnated wipe after each use and store dry. On discharge, wash with detergent, immerse in 70% alcohol for 10 minutes. Wipe and store dry.	*Communal thermometers:* wipe clean, wash in a cold neutral detergent, rinse, dry and immerse in 70% isopropyl alcohol for 10 minutes. Wipe and store dry.
Thermometers (rectal)	Wash in detergent solution after each use, wipe dry and immerse in 70% alcohol for 10 minutes. Wipe and store dry.	
Toilet seats	Wash daily with detergent and dry.	*Infected patients or if grossly contaminated:* Wash with disinfectant solution, rinse and dry. This is important in an area where soiling is more likely, ie Gynaecology, Maternity, Urology Department, etc.
Tooth mugs	Use disposable.	Heat disinfect in CSSD, if non-disposable.
Toys	*Soft toys:* machine wash, rinse and dry thoroughly. Do not soak toys in a disinfectant solution. *Others:* wash with detergent, rinse and dry or wipe with an alcohol impregnated swab.	For children with infectious diseases do not use communal toys or those which cannot easily be disinfected. Heavily contaminated soft toys may have to be destroyed.
Trolleys	Wash trolley and wheels daily with detergent, rinse and dry at beginning of dressing round only.	Wipe trolley tops with an alcohol impregnated wipe before and after use. If contaminated, clean first, then use an alcohol impregnated wipe.

Table 3.5 – Continued

Equipment or site	Routine or preferred method	Acceptable alternative or additional recommendations
Tubing (anaesthetic or ventilator)	Reprocess by washing and sterilization in CSSD,	*Infected patients:* For patient with respiratory infection, tuberculosis or patients with AIDS use disposable tubing. *Never* use glutaraldehyde to disinfect respiratory equipment.
Ultrasound	Disinfect ultrasound head with 70% isopropyl alcohol between each patient.	
Urinals	Heat disinfect in a bedpan washer at a temperature of 80°C for 1 minute or use disposables.	Disposable urinals must be disposed of in a macerator unit.
Ventilators	Cleaning and disinfecting this equipment is a procedure which is normally carried out in a specified area (ie ICU, SCBU, CSSD) according to written protocol based on manufacturer's recommendations.	Contact a member of the Infection Control Team for advice if required.
Wash basins/sink	Clean with detergent, use cream cleaner for stains, scum etc. Disinfection is not normally required.	Disinfection may be required if contaminated. Use non-abrasive hypochlorite powder or hypochlorite/detergent solution.
X-ray equipment	Damp dust with detergent solution, do not over-wet, and allow surface to dry before use.	Clean with detergent and then wipe with an alcohol impregnated wipe to disinfect. For specialised equipment, draw up local protocol for cleaning and disinfection, based on the manufacturer's recommendations.

References and further reading

Department of Health. *Sterilization, Disinfection and Cleaning of Medical Equipment: guidance on decontamination from the Microbiology Advisory Committee to Department of Health Medical Devices Directorate.* Part 1 *Principles.* London: Medical Devices Agency, 1993.

Department of Health. *Sterilization, Disinfection and Cleaning of Medical Equipment: guidance on decontamination from the Microbiology Advisory Committee to Department of Health Medical Devices Directorate.* Part 2 *Protocols.* London: Medical Devices Agency, 1996.

Ayliffe GAJ, Coates D, Hoffman PN. *Chemical Disinfection in Hospitals.* 2nd ed. London: Public Health Laboratory Service, 1993.

Larson E, Faan RN. Guideline for use of topical antimicrobial agents. *American Journal of Infection* 1988; **16(6):** 253-266.

Coates D, Hutchinson DN. How to produce disinfection policy. *Journal of Hospital Infection* 1994;**26:**57-68.

Rutala WA. APIC guideline for selection and use of disinfectants. *American Journal of Infection Control* 1996; **24(4)** Suppl: 313-342.

Favero MS, Bond WW. Chemical disinfection of medical and surgical materials. In: Block SS, ed. *Disinfection, sterilization and preservation.* 4th ed. Philadelphia: Lea and Febiger, 1991: 617-641.

British Society of Gastroenterology. Cleaning and disinfection of equipment for gastrointestinal flexible endoscopy: interim recommendations of a working party of the British Society of Gastroenterology. *Gut,* 1988; **29:** 1134-1151(under revision).

Cooke RP *et al.* Decontamination of urological equipment: interim report of a working group of the Standing Committee on the Urological Equipment of the British Association of Urological Surgeon. *British Journal of Urology,* 1993; **71:** 5-9.

Woodcock *et al.* Bronchoscopy and infection control. *Lancet,* 1989;**2:** 270-271.

Ayliffe GAJ, Babb JR, Bradley CR. Sterilization of arthroscopes and laparoscopes. *Journal of Hospital Infection* 1992; **22:** 265-269.

Axon ATR. Working Party Report to the World Congresses of Gastroenterology, Sydney 1990. Disinfection and endoscopes: Summary and recommendations. *Journal of Gastroenterology and Hepatology* 1990;**6:**23-24.

Martin MA, Reichelderfer M. APIC guideline for infection prevention and control in flexible endoscopy. *American Journal of Infection Control* 1994; **22(1):** 19-38.

Department of Health. *Decontamination of endoscopes.* London: Medical Devices Agency, 1996.

4

PREVENTION OF INFECTION CAUSED BY SPECIFIC PATHOGENS

METHICILLIN RESISTANT *STAPHYLOCOCCUS AUREUS*

Staphylococcus aureus is one of the most common pathogens well known for causing skin and soft tissue infection. Up to 30% of healthy people carry *Staph.aureus* in their nose and other moist or hairy body areas. The majority of these are sensitive to commonly used antibiotics. Methicillin (Flucloxacillin) resistant *Staphylococcus aureus* (MRSA) are important in that they are resistant to flucloxacillin and erythromycin, the most commonly used antibiotics to treat *Staph.aureus* infection, but they are also resistant to other antibiotics, leaving only glycopeptides, eg vancomycin or teicoplanin for treatment which has to be given intravenously, are potentially toxic and expensive. The consequence of not controlling MRSA in hospitals could lead to increased cost because of increased length of stay of patients in hospital and increased cost of glycopeptide antibiotics for treatment.

There are many different strains of MRSA, some of which may be Epidemic in character, causing serious outbreaks and they are called EMRSA; in general they are of equivalent pathogenicity to ordinary *Staph.aureus*.

Management in hospital

All patients known to be infected or colonized with MRSA should be admitted directly to a single room with contact isolation precautions (see page 26). A member of the Infection Control Team should be notified when admission is planned or occurs. In some situations where there is more than one patient with MRSA it may be possible to cohort the patients into one suitable area or unit which should be done on the advice of Infection Control Team. The patient should be promptly discharged from hospital if the clinical condition allows.

All patients admitted from other hospitals and patients from other countries requiring medical treatment, especially if they have a history of previous hospital admission, should be admitted to a side ward and screened for carriage of MRSA. If the specimens are sent to the microbiology laboratory then request forms should include information on MRSA status and screening swabs should be sent marked "MRSA screening swabs". All patients admitted to the ward from the elderly unit should also be isolated in a side ward and screened on admission according to local protocol. If the screening swabs are clear then they should be transferred to an open ward. If the screened swabs are positive then they should be kept in a side ward. The patient's case notes must be identified with a warning MRSA sticker. They should also be "flagged" on the Patient Information Services (PIS) computer, if possible.

MRSA

ISOLATE ON ADMISSION

CONTACT
INFECTION CONTROL NURSE
or **INFECTION CONTROL DOCTOR**

If the patient requires treatment in another hospital the clinician and the Infection Control Team at the receiving hospital *must* be informed.

Infection control precautions

- Isolate all known cases of MRSA in a single room with contact isolation precautions (see page 26) or cohort the patients into a suitable area of ward or unit. The patient may not leave the room without consultation with the nurse-in-charge.

- The number of staff caring for the patient should be kept to a minimum, if possible. Staff with skin lesions, eczema or superficial skin sepsis must be excluded from contact with the patient.

- Single-use disposable latex gloves must be worn for handling contaminated tissue, dressings or linen. Hands must be washed after removing gloves. Single-use disposable plastic aprons must be worn for activities involving contact with the patient or their environment. Used plastic aprons should be discarded into a yellow clinical waste bag before leaving the room. For extensive physical contact with the patient, non-permeable disposable gowns are required. High efficiency filter type masks should be worn for procedures that may generate

Staphylococcus aerosols, eg sputum suction, chest physiotherapy or procedures on patients with an exfoliative skin condition, and when performing dressings on patients with extensive burns or lesions.

- Hands must be washed before and after contact with the patient or their immediate environment. They should be washed thoroughly using an antiseptic chlorhexidine/detergent ("Hibiscrub") or alternatively, physically clean hands can be treated with an alcoholic ("Hibisol") hand rub.

- All single-use items must be disposed of as clinical waste. Clinical waste bags must be sealed before leaving the room. Any re-usable items must be processed in accordance with the local disinfection policy.

- Used linen must be handled gently at all times. All bed linen and clothing must be changed daily. Linen must be processed as infected linen according to the local policy. The linen bags must be sealed at the bedside and removed directly to the dirty utility area or to the collection point.

- The room should be cleaned after all other areas of the ward. A freshly prepared hypochlorite (1,000 ppm av Cl_2) disinfectant should be used.

Visits to other departments

- Visits by patients with MRSA to other departments should be kept to a minimum.

- For any treatment or investigations, prior arrangements must be made with the senior staff of the department concerned. They should be seen immediately and not left in a waiting room with other patients. The Infection Control Team will advise on the necessary infection control precautions.

- The patient should be seen or treated at the end of the working session and spend the minimum time in the department.

- Clearance of MRSA carriage should be attempted before surgery wherever possible. These patients should be operated upon at the end of an operating list. All lesions must be covered with an impermeable dressing during the operation and the adjacent areas treated with appropriate antiseptic.

- Prophylactic vancomycin or teicoplanin should be considered for colonized or infected patients undergoing surgery or any other invasive procedures. Seek advice from the medical microbiologist.

Transfer of patients

Within the hospital : Transfer of infected or colonized patients to other wards or departments must be kept to the minimum and only after consultation with a member of the Infection Control Team. If the patient must be moved to a different ward, they should, if possible, be bathed with chlorhexidine skin cleanser shampoo. The patient should be given clean clothing and transferred to a clean bed. All open lesions must be covered with an impermeable dressing during the transfer.

To other hospitals: Inter-hospital movement should be restricted where this is possible. It is the responsibility of the clinician-in-charge of the patient to inform the clinician of the receiving hospital about the patient's MRSA status. Inform a member of the local Infection Control Team about such a transfer who will liaise with a member of the Infection Control Team at the receiving hospital. A letter should also be sent giving the relevant clinical details as to whether the patient is infected or colonized with MRSA and the details of the treatment protocol, so that a course of treatment can be completed.

Nursing or residential home: Continued carriage of MRSA is not a contraindication for the transfer of the patient to a nursing or residential home. If the patient is discharged to the residential or nursing home, the clinician should inform the general practitioner, owner of the nursing home and other health care agencies involved in the patient's management. A discharge letter should be sent which includes a copy of decontamination protocol so that the course of treatment is completed. A member of the Infection Control Team should also be informed in the usual way. The Consultant in Communicable Disease Control should also be informed about such a transfer.

The patient should be advised that there is no risk to healthy relatives or others outside the hospital, unless they are hospital workers with patient contact. In such cases, the health care worker who has been in contact should notify the Occupational Health Department and the Infection Control Doctor. All the patients should be given the fact sheet about MRSA.

Ambulance transportation

The ambulance service must be notified in advance. There is no evidence that ambulance staff or their families are at risk from transporting patients with MRSA. The following infection control measures should be taken by the ambulance staff to minimize the risk to other ambulance patients who may be at risk of acquiring MRSA.

- The patient should be given clean clothing before transport.
- Wear a disposable plastic apron for contact with the patient.

- Minimize patient contact where this is possible.
- Physically clean hands can be treated with a 3-5 ml application of an alcoholic hand rub ("Hibisol") containing emollient, after contact with the patient or their environment.
- The local area of patient contact, such as the chair and stretcher, should be cleaned with freshly prepared hypochlorite (1000 ppm av Cl_2) solution or with a large alcohol impregnated wipe after transporting an affected patient.
- Blankets and pillow cases must be placed in a water soluble bag then in a red plastic bag and processed as infected linen according to the local policy.
- The ambulance vehicle should be thoroughly cleaned with freshly prepared hypochlorite (1000 ppm av Cl_2) disinfectant and may be used when all surfaces are dry. Fumigation and prolonged airing are not necessary. Once the ambulance is dry it can be used for other patients.

Health care worker

There is no evidence that MRSA poses a risk to healthy people. This includes health care workers and their families. However, where it is indicated, the Occupational Health Department will be involved in the assessment, screening and treatment of staff on the advice of the Infection Control Doctor. The Occupational Health Department will notify the health care worker's general practitioner.

It is the responsibility of all health care workers who have worked in hospital or health care facility where MRSA was endemic, or they have reason to believe that they may be carriers of MRSA, to inform the Occupational Health Department before commencing their employment.

Patient screening

A swab moistened with sterile water should be used to sample carrier sites and lesions. The screening swabs should be taken from nose, perineum/groin, operative & wound sites, abnormal or damaged skin, insertion sites of IV lines, catheter urine samples and sputum, if expectorating. The results of screening swabs are normally available in 3-4 days.

If asymptomatic patients are found to be carriers of MRSA, it is worthwhile discharging them from hospital (if clinical condition permits) on an anti-staphylococcal protocol for elimination of MRSA to reduce the reservoir of MRSA in the community, which in turn will minimize the number of MRSA patients being admitted to the hospital from the community.

Treatment of carriage

Treatment will be prescribed by a medical practitioner on an individual basis, usually in consultation with the medical microbiologist/Infection Control Doctor. The following are general guidelines:

Nares: Apply 2% mupirocin ("Bactroban" nasal) three times a day for 7 days. A small amount of ointment (about the size of a match-head) should be placed on a cotton bud or on the little finger and applied to the anterior part of the inside of each nostril. The nostrils are closed by pressing the sides of the nose together; this will spread the ointment throughout the nares. A cotton bud should be used instead of the little finger for application, especially to infants and patients who are very ill.

Body Bath: *Shower:* Shower with an antiseptic (chlorhexidine, or triclosan) can be used. Apply antiseptic solution beginning with the face and working downwards, paying particular attention to areas around the nose, axillae, umbilicus, groin and perineum. The body is then rinsed and the wash repeated, this time including the hair. Finally, the patient rinses their entire body thoroughly and dries with a clean towel.

Bath: Add an antiseptic (chlorhexidine, triclosan) bath concentrate to a bath full of water immediately prior to the patients entering the water.

Body wash: Patients confined to bed can be washed with an antiseptic (chlorhexidine, triclosan) which can be applied directly after the body is wet, using a standard bed bath technique.

Axillae and perineum: Hexachlorophane 0.33% powder ("Ster-Zac" powder) can be used to treat carrier sites. It should be applied to intact skin such as perineum, buttocks, flexures and axillae for 5 days. ***Do not*** use hexachlorophane powder on badly excoriated or inflamed skin or during pregnancy. The product should be administered to children under two years of age on medical advice only.

Colonized Lesions: 2% mupirocin ("Bactroban ointment") can be applied topically three times a day to colonized lesion for 7 days. Topical preparation contains polyethylene glycol which can be absorbed from open wounds and damages skin and is excreted by kidneys. Therefore, it should be used with caution if there is evidence of moderate or severe renal impairment.

Antiseptic detergents should be used with care in patients with dermatitis and broken skin and ***must*** be discontinued if skin irritation develops.

Topical nasal applications are usually ineffective in clearing throat or sputum colonization. It is also often difficult to eradicate colonization from chronic lesions such as pressure sores or leg ulcers in elderly patients. In these situations, reliance must be placed on isolation procedures and early discharge. Systematic therapy can be given as advised by the medical microbiologist on an individual patient basis.

It is important that patients' clothes should be changed daily and washed in a hot water cycle. Dry clean non-washable and woollen clothes. Bed linen should be changed at the beginning of protocol and then every day until the end of protocol. Soft personal items should be washed in hot cycle or dry clean at the beginning of protocol.

Microbiological surveillance

Once the patient is positive for MRSA, swabs from carrier and other sites should be taken at least 5 days after stopping MRSA treatment protocol. Three sets of negative screening swabs are required before the patient is considered to be "clear", as scanty colonization may not be detected with fewer screening specimens.

Follow-up screening swabs will be advised by a member of the Infection Control Team. Relapses may occur and prolonged treatment may be required. Relapses are particularly likely if the patient is receiving antibiotics and can occur after relatively long periods, such as 6-12 months. Carriage of MRSA strains may persist for months or years and may reappear in an apparently "clear or cured" patient.

References and further reading

Report of a Combined Working Party of the Hospital Infection Society and the British Society of Antimicrobial Chemotherapy. Revised guidelines for the control of epidemic methicillin-resistant *Staphylococcus aureus*. *Journal of Hospital Infection* 1990; **16:** 351-377 (under revision).

Report of a Combined Working Party of the British Society for Antimicrobial Chemotherapy and the Hospital Infection Society. Guidelines on the control of methicillin-resistant *Staphylococcus aureus* in the community. *Journal of Hospital Infection* 1995; **31:** 1-12.

Duckworth GJ. Diagnosis and management of methicillin resistant *Staphylococcus aureus* infection. *British Medical Journal* 1993; **307:** 1049-1052.

Cafferkey MT, ed. *Methicillin-resistant Staphylococcus aureus: Clinical Management and Laboratory Aspects* New York: Marcel Dekker, 1992.

MENINGOCOCCAL INFECTIONS

Meningococcal disease is caused by *N. meningitidis* or meningococci. They are Gram-negative diplococci which are divided into antigenically distinct groups. The commonest groups are B, C, A, Y and W135. They can cause meningitis and septicaemia. Septicaemia without meningitis has the highest case fatality of 15-20% or more, whereas in meningitis alone the fatality rate is around 3-5%. Most cases are a combination of septicaemia and meningitis.

The disease can affect any age group, but the young are the most vulnerable. Cases occur in all months of the year but the incidence is highest in winter. The nasopharyngeal carriage rate of all meningococci in the general population is about 10%, although rates vary with age; about 25% of young adults may be carriers at any one time.

Person-to-person transmission is mainly by droplets spread from the upper respiratory tract. There is no reservoir other than humans and the organism dies quickly outside the host. The incubation period is 2-10 days but most invasive disease normally develops within seven days of acquisition. Therefore, for practical purposes a one week period is considered sufficient to identify close contacts for prophylaxis. The incubation period is two to three days, and the onset of disease varies from fulminant to insidious with mild prodromal symptoms. Early symptoms and signs are usually malaise, pyrexia and vomiting. Headache, photophobia, drowsiness or confusion, joint pains and a typical haemorrhagic rash of meningococcal septicaemia may develop. Early on, the rash may be non-specific. The rash, which may be petechial or purpuric, does not blanche and this can be confirmed readily by gentle pressure with a glass slide etc, when the rash can be seen to persist. Patients may present in coma. In young infants particularly, the onset may be insidious and the classical signs are absent. The diagnosis should be suspected in the presence of vomiting, pyrexia, irritability and, if still patent, raised anterior fontanelle tension. The guidelines given in this section are based on the recommendations made by the PHLS Meningococcal Infection Working Group and Public Health Medicine Environmental Group.

Emergency action

Urgent admission to the hospital is a priority in view of the potentially rapid clinical progression of meningococcal disease. Early treatment with benzylpenicillin is recommended and may save life. Therefore, all general practitioners should carry benzylpenicillin in their emergency bags and give it while arranging the transfer of the case to the hospital. The only contraindication is a history of penicillin anaphylaxis. In these instances chloramphenicol (1.2 gram for adult; 25 mg/kg for children under age of 12 years) may be given by injection. Immediate dose of benzylpenicillin for suspected cases are:

Adults and children (10 years or over)	1200 mg
Children aged 1-9 years	600 mg
Children aged under 1 year	300 mg

This dose should be given as soon as possible, ideally by intravenous injection. Intramuscular injection is likely to be less effective in shocked patients, due to reduced perfusion, but can be used if vein cannot be found.

Management in hospital

On arrival in the hospital of a suspected case, doctors should take blood for culture and give benzylpenicillin (or suitable alternative) immediately if this has not already been done.

All patients with known or suspected meningitis must be isolated in a single room at the time of admission, with respiratory isolation precautions (see page 23). The patient should be isolated for a *minimum* of 48 hours after the start of appropriate antibiotic and a full course of chemoprophylaxis has been given.

Laboratory investigations

- Blood for culture on all cases.
- Cerebrospinal fluid (CSF) for direct microscopy and culture. Lumber puncture should only be done *if there are no clinical contraindications*.
- Throat swabs (a sweep of the pharyngeal wall and tonsils) from all patients. If this is impossible, eg from a baby or uncooperative patient, a pernasal swab rotated on the posterior pharyngeal wall is taken as an alternative, as the organism can often be cultured from these sites despite pre-admission antibiotics.
- If the patient has a haemorrhagic skin rash (petechiae, purpura, or larger area of haemorrhage) lesions can be aspirated or swabbed for microscopy and culture.
- CSF and blood (2.5 ml EDTA or citrated specimens) should be taken on admission for polymerase chain reaction (PCR).
- Paired serum sample (at least 0.5-1ml) should be sent for meningococcal antibodies; first (acute) sample should be taken at the time of admission and second (convalescent) sample taken between 2-6 weeks after hospital admission.
- Other laboratory investigations should be done as clinically indicated.

Notification

Meningococcal disease is a notifiable disease, therefore all known or suspected cases of *N. meningitidis* infection must be notified immediately by telephone (followed by written confirmation) to the local Consultant in Communicable Disease Control (CCDC) who will co-ordinate chemoprophylaxis and immunization where appropriate. If the CCDC receive a delayed report of a case, household contacts should be offered chemoprophylaxis and vaccine, if appropriate, up to four weeks after the index case became ill.

Chemoprophylaxis

Although penicillin and cefotaxime are the drugs of choice for the treatment of meningococcal infection, they have no effect on the elimination of nasopharyngeal carriage of the organism and are therefore not indicated for prophylaxis. Rifampicin, ciprofloxacin and ceftriaxone are effective in reducing the nasopharyngeal carriage rate and are therefore recommended for chemoprophylaxis.

Rifampicin: In the absence of contraindications, the drug of choice is rifampicin, which can be used in all age groups. It should preferably be taken at least 30 minutes before a meal or 2 hours after a meal to ensure rapid and complete absorption. Dosages of rifampicin are as follows:

Adults:	600 mg every 12 hours for 2 days.
Children:	
– (Over 1 year)	10 mg/kg every 12 hours for 2 days (up to a maximum of 600 mg per dose).
– (3 months to 1 year)	5 mg/kg every 12 hours for 2 days.

Rifampicin is contraindicated in the presence of jaundice or known hypersensitivity to rifampicin. Interactions with other drugs, such as anticoagulants, should be considered. It also interferes with hormonal contraceptives (family planning association advice for a "missed" pill should be followed if rifampicin is prescribed to an oral contraceptive user) and causes red coloration of urine, sputum and tears, (soft contact lenses may be permanently stained). Side effects should be explained to the patients and the information should be supplied with the prescription.

Ciprofloxacin: Ciprofloxacin ("Ciproxin") can be offered as an alternative to rifampicin and is given as a single dose of 500 mg orally *in adults* (not licensed for this purpose). It is useful when large numbers of contacts need prophylaxis, such as in the management of outbreaks in colleges or military camps or where compliance is in doubt.

Ceftriaxone: Although no drug is considered to be safe in pregnancy, all pregnant women who are contacts should be counselled carefully about risks and benefits and the option to give prophylaxis should be discussed. Ceftriaxone ("Rocephein") can be given as a first choice in pregnancy. It can also be used as an alternative to rifampicin or where compliance is in doubt. dosages of ceftriaxone are:

Adults: A single dose of 250 mg intramuscular injection.

Children: A single dose of 125 mg intramuscular injection (from 6 weeks to 12 years).

Ceftriaxone is contraindicated in patients with a history of hypersensitivity to cephalosporins. It is not recommended for premature infants and full-term infants during the first six weeks of life.

Management of contacts

Public health action is indicated for confirmed and probable cases but not in response to possible cases. The following case definitions are defined by the PHLS meningococcal working group :

Confirmed Case: Clinical diagnosis of meningitis or septicaemia confirmed microbiologically as caused by *Neisseria meningitidis*. Meningococcal infection of joint, heart, or eye (including conjunctiva), should also be regarded as a confirmed case for public health action.

Probable case: Clinical diagnosis of meningococcal meningitis or septicaemia without microbiological confirmation in which the CCDC, in consultation with the clinician managing the case, considers that meningococcal disease is the likeliest diagnosis. In the absence of an alternative diagnosis a feverish, ill patient with a petechial/purpuric rash should be regarded as a probable case of meningococcal septicaemia.

Possible case: As probable case, but the CCDC, in consultation with the clinician managing the case, considers that diagnoses other than meningococcal disease are at least as likely. This category includes cases treated with antibiotics whose probable diagnosis is viral meningitis.

After single case

Chemoprophylaxis should be offered to all close contacts (defined as people who had *close, prolonged contact* with the case) as soon as possible, ie within 24 hours after the diagnosis of index case. Prophylaxis is recommended to the contacts of confirmed or probable cases 7 days before the case became ill. Contacts of possible cases do not need prophylaxis unless or until further evidence emerges that changes the diagnostic category to confirmed or probable. It is recommended in the following situations:

Household: Immediate family and close contacts, ie people sleeping in the same house and boy/girl friends as the index case.

Kissing: Those people who have been mouth kissing contacts with the index case.

Index case: Index case should receive prophylaxis (unless they have already been treated with ceftriaxone) as soon as they are able to take oral medication.

Health care worker: Health care workers who have been involved in mouth-to-mouth resuscitation with meningitis case.

Cluster of cases

A cluster is defined as two or more cases of meningococcal disease in the same preschool group, school, or college/university within a four week period. If two possible cases attend the same institution, whatever the interval between cases, prophylaxis to household or institutional contacts is not indicated.

If two confirmed cases caused by different serogroups attend the same institution, they should be regarded as two sporadic cases, whatever the interval between them. Only household contacts of each case should be offered prophylaxis.

If two confirmed or probable cases who attend the same preschool group or school arise within a four week period and are, or could be, caused by the same serogroup, wider public health action in the institution is usually indicated.

The principle of managing such clusters is to attempt to define a group at high risk of acquiring meningococcal infection and disease, and to target that group for public health action. The target group should be a discrete group that contains the cases and makes sense to staff and parents, eg children and staff of the same preschool group, children of the same school year, children who share a common social activity, or a group of friends. Management of clusters should be decided by the CCDC who should seek advice from the appropriate experts.

It is important to emphasize that chemoprophylaxis is effective in reducing the nasopharyngeal carriage rates after treatment but *does not* completely eliminate transmission between household members. Contacts should be reminded of the persisting risk of disease, whether or not prophylaxis is given, and of the need to contact their general practitioner urgently if they develop any symptoms suggestive of meningococcal disease.

Immunisation of contacts

Close contacts of cases of meningococcal meningitis have a considerably increased risk of developing the disease in the subsequent months, despite appropriate chemoprophylaxis. Therefore, immediate family or close contacts of cases of group A or group C meningitis should be given meningococcal vaccine in addition to chemoprophylaxis. The latter should be given first and the decision to offer vaccine should be made when the results of typing are available. *Vaccine should not be given to contacts of group B cases.* The serological response is detected in more than 90% of recipients and occurs 5-7 days after a single injection. The response is strictly group specific and confers no protection against group B organisms. If the causative organism is identified as a group A or C, meningococcal vaccination (a single dose of 0.5 ml is given by deep subcutaneous intramuscular injection in adults and children from 2 months of age) should be offered to the close contacts.

Further information can be obtained from PHLS Meningococcal Reference Unit, Manchester, telephone 0161 445 2416; Gloucester Public Health Laboratory, Gloucester, telephone 01452 305334; PHLS Communicable Disease Surveillance Centre, London. telephone 0181 200 6868; Scottish Centre for Infection and Environmental Health, telephone 0141 946 7120 or Scottish Meningococcal and Pneumococcal Reference Laboratory, telephone 0141 201 3836.

References and further reading

PHLS Meningococcal Infection Working Party and Public Health Medicine Environmental Group. Control of meningococcal disease: guidance for consultants in communicable disease control. *Communicable Disease Report* 1995; **5:** R189-195.

Kaczmarski EB, Cartwright KAV. Control of meningococcal disease: guidance for microbiologist. *Communicable Disease Report* 1995; **5:** R196-198.

PHLS Meningococcus Working Group and Public Health Medicine Environmental Group. Management of clusters of meningococcal disease. *Communicable Disease Report* 1997; **7:** R3-5.

Department of Health, Welsh Office, Scottish Office Department of Health, DHSS (N. Ireland). *Immunization against infectious diseases* London: HMSO, 1996.

Hart CA, Rogers TRF, eds. Meningococcal disease. *Journal of Medical Microbiology* 1993; **39:**2-25.

Cartwright K, ed. *Meningococcal Disease* London: Wiley, 1995.

GASTROINTESTINAL INFECTIONS AND FOOD POISONING

Diarrhoea and vomiting may be caused by many agents, both infective and non-infective. The World Health Organization defined food poisoning as *any disease of an infectious or toxic nature caused by or thought to be caused by the consumption of food or water.*

All cases of gastroenteritis should be regarded as potentially infectious until appropriate investigations is completed. In hospital, they should be isolated in a single room with enteric isolation precaution (see page 27) and must be reported immediately to a member of the Infection Control Team; the Consultant in Communicable Diseases Control (CCDC) should also be informed. In the community, it is the responsibility of the general practitioner to report all communicable diseases and episodes of gastroenteritis to the CCDC who will assess the situation and implement control measures, if necessary.

Persons in occupations or circumstances where there is a special risk of spreading gastrointestinal infection are defined in four groups defined by the working party of the PHLS Salmonella Committee:

Group 1:   food handlers,

Group 2:   staff in health care facilities,

Group 3:   children < 5 years of age, and

Group 4:   older children and adults who may find it difficult to implement good standards of personal hygiene.

It is normal practice to exclude a patient with gastroenteritis from work or school until the person is free of diarrhoea and vomiting and, if necessary, the appropriate clearance tests have been completed. Thereafter, it is particularly important to assess the risk of spreading infection in the four groups of persons in whom special action should be considered. The circumstances of each case, excreter, carrier or contact in these groups, should be considered individually and factors such as standards of personal hygiene should be taken into account. It is important to emphasize that the agents causing gastroenteritis may infect without causing symptoms or be excreted for long periods after recovery from clinical illness. Excretion of organisms may still occur intermittently and in small numbers. Under these circumstances transmission is unlikely providing that good personal hygiene is practised.

Members of staff suffering from gastrointestinal or food poisoning infection should inform the manager who will notify the Occupational Health Department. If the member of staff works in the kitchen or an area where food and enteral feed are prepared or handled, the catering manager and a member of the Infection Control Team should be informed.

All suspected outbreaks of gasterointestinal infection among staff and patients in the hospital must be reported to the Infection Control Doctor and the Infection Control Nurse as a matter of urgency, who will investigate the incident and liaise with the CCDC.

References and further reading

The prevention of human transmission of gastrointestinal infections, infestations, and bacterial intoxication. A guide for Public Health Physicians and Environmental Health Officers in England and Wales. A Working Party of the PHLS Salmonella sub-committee. *Communicable Disease Report* 1995; **5:** R158-172.

Department of Health. *Management of outbreaks of foodborne illness* London: Department of Health,1994.

Scottish Home and Health Department. *The investigation and control of foodborne and waterborne diseases in Scotland* Edinburgh: HMSO, 1995.

Consultants in Public Health Medicine (Communicable Disease and Environmental Health Working Group). Scottish Centre for Infection and Environmental Health. Guidelines for bacteriological clearance following gastroenteritic infection. *Communicable Disease (Scotland) Weekly Report* 1994; **28(26):** 8-13.

PHLS Working Group on the Control of *Shigella sonnei.* Revised Guidelines for the control *Shigella sonnei* infection and other infective diarrhoeas. *Communicable Disease Report* 1993; **5:** R69-70.

Subcommittee of the PHLS Working Group on the Vero-cytotoxin producing *Escherichia coli* (VTEC). Interim guidelines for the control if infections with Vero cyto-toxin producing *Escherichia coli* (VTEC). *Communicable Disease Report* 1995; **6**: R77-81.

TUBERCULOSIS

Tuberculosis is an infection caused by bacterium of the *Mycobacterium tuberculosis* complex (*M.tuberculosis, M.bovis, M.africanum*) which may affect any part of the body, but most commonly affects the lungs and the lymph nodes. In the UK, about three quarters of the cases involve the lungs and infection is usually acquired by inhaling infected droplets coughed by a person with tuberculosis of the lung. Non-respiratory disease is more common in children, in immigrants from countries with a high prevalence of tuberculosis and in people with impaired immunity, (eg patients with AIDS & HIV infection).

Risk factors for acquiring tuberculosis include extremes of age, concomitant HIV infection, ethnic group from high prevalence countries, chronic alcohol misuse, poor socio-economic background and homelessness.

Once the individual has acquired the infection it may heal spontaneously or, over weeks/months, active disease develops. It may be contained and unapparent at the time but may cause active disease (reactivation) later in life because of old age or other events that weaken the individual's immunity.

The treatment of tuberculosis is complex and lengthy and requires close supervision and specialist knowledge beyond the scope of this book. In the UK, guidance on the treatment of tuberculosis is based on the recommendations of the British Thoracic Society protocols. Most patients with tuberculosis can be treated at home; a few require hospital admission for severe illness, adverse effects of chemotherapy, or for social reasons.

Infection control precautions

- All suspected or confirmed (sputum smear [AAFB] positive) patients, including those previously negative who become smear positive on or after bronchoscopy, should be isolated in a single room with the infection control measures outlined under respiratory isolation precautions (see page 23).

- Adult patients with pulmonary TB with three negative smear samples and patients with non-pulmonary TB (with the exception of those with infected discharging wounds) should be regarded as non-infectious and may be nursed in a general ward.

- No patient with suspected or confirmed respiratory tuberculosis, whatever the sputum status, should be admitted to an open ward containing immunocompromised patients, such as HIV infected, transplant or oncology patients, until pronounced non-infectious by the physician-in-charge in consultation with the Infection Control Doctor because of the known possibility of transmission of infection from and to HIV infected patients and the seriousness of multidrug resistant tuberculosis. Cough inducing procedures such as inhalation of pentamidine, or for production of sputum, should never be performed in an open ward or bay and appropriate environmental controls should be in place.

- The patient should be isolated in a single room with negative pressure airflow ventilation in relation to the surrounding area; air should be mechanically extracted (without recirculation) to the outside, away from patient areas and inlets for air conditioning. The door should be kept closed as much as possible.

- Patients in isolation should not visit wards, including communal washing facilities, or public areas of the hospital and should not walk or be transported through open wards which may contain immuno-compromised patients, unless they are wearing a mask.

- All patients should be informed that their infection is spread to others by the respiratory route. Routine surgical masks are recommended for patients with uncontrolled cough or sneezing to reduce aerosol generation. Other patients should be taught to cover the mouth and nose with disposable paper tissue whilst coughing and to dispose of the tissue in a clinical waste bin.

- Wearing of a mask for staff is recommended when direct exposure to respiratory secretions is unavoidable, eg during bronchoscopy or prolonged care of a high dependency patient, after cough inducing procedures or when performing the last offices. A high efficiency particulate air (HEPA) mask should be used. Masks should be close fitting and filter particles of 1-5 microns. Use of a mask is not a substitute for good infection control management.

- Visitors should, as far as possible, be limited to those who have already been in close contact before the diagnosis. Contact with staff should be kept to a reasonable minimum without compromising patient care.

- All children with tuberculosis and their visitors should be segregated from other patients until the contacts have been screened and pronounced non-infectious. It is possible that one of the visitors may have been the source of the child's infection and hence be a risk to other patients if the child is in an open ward.

- If there is any doubt about the degree of isolation required, the case should be discussed with the Infection Control Team who should also be informed of any sputum smear positive patient in the hospital.

- Termination of isolation should be decided by the physician-in-charge in conjunction with the Infection Control Doctor. Uncomplicated sputum positive tuberculosis will usually be non-infectious after two weeks compliant with standard multidrug chemotherapy and the patient may then be transferred to an open ward, but the results of any sputum tests and/or response to treatment should be taken into account.

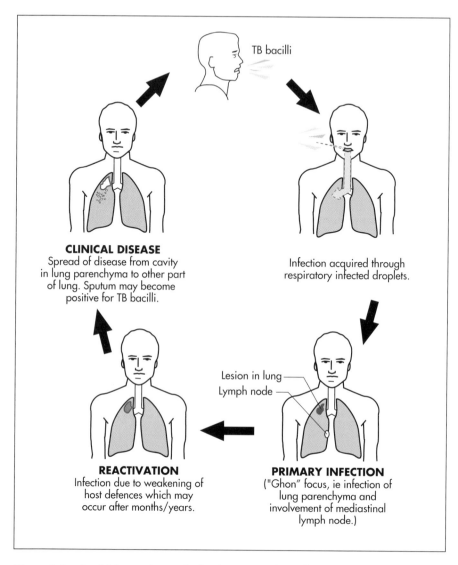

Figure 4.1 – Aquisition and spread of pulmonary tuberculosis.

Multidrug resistant tuberculosis

Multidrug resistant tuberculosis (MDR-TB) is, by definition, tuberculosis resistant to two or more of the main line anti-tuberculosis drugs (usually isoniazid and rifampicin with or without other drugs). The implication is serious both for the individual and for the public health because of the limited number of the alternative anti-tuberculosis drugs available for treatment. Additional precautions may be required for patients with MDR-TB which should be considered on a case by case basis with the discussion of Infection Control Doctor. Drug resistant disease should be considered when there is:

- a history of previous incomplete or non-compliant treatment.
- contact with a patient with known drug resistant disease.
- disease probably acquired in a country with high incidence of drug resistance.
- disease not responding to treatment.

Contact tracing

Contact tracing is an integral part of the routine management of patients with tuberculosis and should be limited in the first instance to close contacts, ie household and close associates of patients with respiratory tuberculosis. If initial investigation reveals a number of contacts with evidence of tuberculosis, consideration should be given to widening the circle of contacts who may be offered screening. The person responsible for local contact tracing should be named in the hospital policy.

- Contacts should only be considered significant if the source is smear positive on direct sputum examination or on examination of bronchial washings.

- Staff undertaking mouth-to-mouth resuscitation, prolonged care of a high dependency patient or repeated chest physiotherapy should be considered as close contacts.

- All members of staff should be seen in the Occupational Health Department and have their occupational health notes reviewed to ascertain whether they have had a Heaf test, BCG vaccination and BCG scar. Enquiries should be made as to any current illness or treatment that might result in their immune system being compromised.

- Those close contacts who have not had previous BCG vaccination should be Heaf tested.

- Those staff with a negative or grade 1 Heaf reaction should be retested two months after the last contact to allow for tuberculin conversion. Staff who are persistently Heaf negative should be offered BCG vaccination. Those who convert to a positive Heaf test should be referred to a respiratory physician.

- Those who have a previous history of BCG vaccination and/or were previously positive on Heaf test, do not require further investigation but should be advised of the possible symptoms of tuberculosis and the importance of reporting such symptoms promptly.

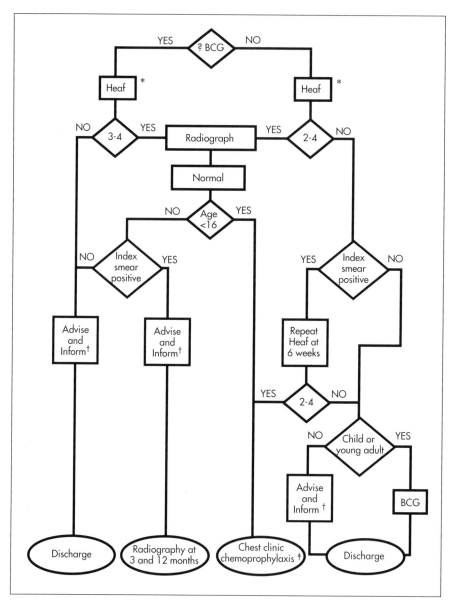

Figure 4.2 – Examination of close contacts of pulmonary tuberculosis. *Note:* children under two who have not had BCG vaccination and who are close contacts of a smear positive adult index patient should recieve chemoprophylaxis irrespective of tuberculin status (plus BCG vaccination later if applicable). *Negative test in immunosuppressed subjects does not exclude tuberculous infection. † Advise patient of tuberculosis symptoms, inform GP of contact. ‡Person eligible for, but not given, chemoprophylaxis should have a chest radiograph at 3 and 12 months.
(Reproduced with permission from the Joint Tuberculosis Committee of the British Thoracic Society. *Thorax* 1994;**49:**1193–1200.)

If a patient in a general ward is diagnosed as having open pulmonary, particularly after a delay of several days, other patients in the ward should have their exposure documented and their consultants should be advised. No action is required unless patients are unusually susceptible to infection or the index case proves to be highly infectious, in which case appropriate examination and follow-up is undertaken.

References and further reading

Department of Health Welsh Office. *The Prevention and Control of Tuberculosis in the United Kingdom: Recommendations for the prevention and control of tuberculosis at local level.* London: Department of Health, 1996.

Department of Health Welsh Office. *The Prevention and Control of Tuberculosis in the United Kingdom: Tuberculosis and homeless people.* London: Department of Health, 1996.

Joint Tuberculosis Committee of the British Thoracic Society. Control and prevention of tuberculosis in the United Kingdom: Code of Practice 1994. *Thorax* 1994; **49:** 1193-1200.

Subcommittee of the Joint Tuberculosis Committee of the British Thoracic Society. Guidelines on the management of tuberculosis and HIV infection in the United Kingdom. *British Medical Journal* 1992; **304:** 1231-1233.

Subcommittee of the Joint Tuberculosis Committee of the British Thoracic Society. Chemotherapy and management of tuberculosis in the United Kingdom: recommendations of the Joint Tuberculosis Committee of the British Thoracic Society. *Thorax* 1990; **45:** 403-408.

Cookson ST, Jarvis WR. Prevention of Nosocomial Transmission of *Mycobactrium tuberculosis*. *Infectious Disease Clinics of North America* 1997; **11(2):** 385-409

VARICELLA/HERPES ZOSTER

Chickenpox (varicella) is an acute, generalized viral disease caused by varicella zoster virus (VZV). The onset of disease is sudden with slight fever, mild constitutional symptoms and a skin eruption that is maculopapular for a few hours, vesicular for 3-4 days, and leaves a granular scab.

Herpes zoster (shingles) is a local manifestation of reactivation of latent varicella infection in the dorsal root ganglia. Vesicles with an erythematous base are restricted to skin areas supplied by sensory nerves of a single associated group of dorsal root ganglia.

In cases of chickenpox the virus is shed from the nasopharynx for up to 5 days before the rash appears, and then from the skin lesions for about 7 days, until the vesicles have dried to form a scab. In shingles, the virus is shed from the skin lesions rather than from the oropharynx, until the lesions have dried to form scabs. Contagiousness may be prolonged in patients with altered immunity. Susceptible individuals should be considered to be infectious 10-21 days following exposure.

Varicella is transmitted from person-to-person by direct contact or through the respiratory (droplet or airborne) route from spread of vesicle fluid, or secretions of the respiratory tract of chickenpox cases, or the vesicle fluid of patients with herpes zoster. It can also be transmitted indirectly through articles freshly soiled by discharges from vesicles and mucous membranes of infected people.

About 5-8 % of the adult population without a history of chickenpox do not have detectable antibody to VZV and are susceptible. Non-immune hospital staff may acquire VZV infection either in the hospital or from hospitalized patients and are at risk of developing chickenpox. Chickenpox in late pregnancy can be particularly severe, therefore pregnant staff who have no clear history of chickenpox must avoid contact with patients and colleagues with VZV infection. Occupational Health Departments are now screening for VZV status routinely. VZV vaccine will be licensed in the U.K. soon and will probably be offered to non-immune health care workers.

The following measures should be considered in the control of VZV infection in health care setting:

- All patients with clinically suspected chickenpox or herpes zoster must be nursed in a side room with respiratory isolation precautions (see page 23). The room should preferably be under negative pressure ventilation. Infected patients may be cohorted together when necessary.

- Patients with varicella infection and susceptible (non-immune) persons exposed within the previous 21 days should not be hospitalized unless absolutely necessary. In-patients who develop varicella and susceptible patients exposed in hospital should be discharged as soon as possible if clinical condition permits.

- Exposed susceptible persons, when they must be hospitalized, should be kept in respiratory isolation from 10 days following their earliest varicella exposure until 21 days after their most recent exposure.

- All staff and high-risk individuals such as non-immune, neonates and the immunodeficient should be protected from exposure. Susceptible personnel should be excluded from all contact with patients on VZV isolation, including patients with localized zoster.

- Exposed susceptible personnel should be excluded from patient care areas beginning 10 days following earliest varicella exposure until 21 days after latest exposure, and up to 28 days if Varicella Zoster Immunoglobulin (VZIG) has been given.

VZIG prophylaxis is recommended in individuals where the clinical condition increases the risk of varicella. The following patients are at risk of developing VZV:

1. **Pregnant women:** The problems of varicella infection during pregnancy relate to both the mother and fetus and also, when infection take place at term to the new born child. At the antenatal booking of the pregnant women, they should be specifically asked about a positive history of chickenpox. If this is positive, the VZV immune status should be checked. If this is negative then the women should be advised of the need to contact the general practitioner if she comes into contact with a case of chickenpox or herpes zoster during her pregnancy who can arrange for the procurement and the administration of VZIG. This should be administered as soon as possible. If the primary varicella occurs during pregnancy the women should be advised of the likelihood of the fetal involvement, with the reference to the stages of the pregnancy that the infection took place and the providers of her antenatal care should be informed.

If the varicella infection occurs ≥ 8 days before delivery, unapparent or mild in-utero infection may occur. If the infection occurs 7 days before to 28 days after delivery, these women run a high risk of severe disseminated infection in the neonate and the intervention with the VZIG is recommended. This should be administered to the mother before delivery and to the neonate after delivery. Varicella in the neonates should also be treated with aciclovir.

2. **Neonates:** Babies born before 30 weeks of gestation or below 1kg should receive VZIG if exposed to varicella irrespective of the immune status of the mother. It is also given to VZV antibody negative infants exposed to chickenpox or herpes zoster in the first 28 days of life. In neonates VZIG is recommended in infants whose mother developed chickenpox (but not herpes zoster) in the period 7 days before to 28 days after delivery.

3. **Patients with poor immunity:** Patients with cancer, especially of lymphoid tissue, patients with leukaemia, organ transplant, AIDS & HIV infection and patients on chemotherapy for malignant disease.

4. **Patients on systemic steroid drugs:** Patients (or parents of children) at risk who use systemic corticosteroids should be advised to take reasonable steps to avoid close contact with chickenpox or herpes zoster and to seek urgent medical attention if exposed to chickenpox. Manifestations of fulminant illness include pneumonia, hepatitis and disseminated intravascular coagulation; rash is not necessary a prominent features. Patients on steroids who are non-immune may require prophylactic cover with VZIG following contact with a patients with chickenpox or shingles.

The following dosage of Varicella Zoster Immunoglobulin (VZIG) are recommended for various age groups:

Age	Dosage
0-5 years	250 mg
6-10 years	500 mg
11-14 years	750 mg
15 years and over	1000 mg

VZIG is given by **intramuscular** injection as soon as possible and not later than 10 days after exposure. It **must not** be given intravenously. If a second exposure occurs after 3 weeks a further dose is required. VZIG does not prevent infection even when given within 72 hours of exposure. However it may attenuate disease if given up to 10 days after exposure. Severe maternal varicella may still occur despite VZIG prophylaxis.

References and further reading

Department of Health, Welsh Office, Scottish Office Department of Health, DHSS (N. Ireland). *Immunization against infectious diseases* London: HMSO, 1996.

Miller E. Varicella-zoster virus. In: Greenough A *et al*, (ed). *Congenital, perinatal and neonatal infections* London: Churchill and Livingstone, 1992: 223-232

CLOSTRIDIUM DIFFICILE INFECTION

In the last two decades, *Clostridium difficile* has been recognised as a major cause of diarrhoea, particularly in the elderly and debilitated patients and patients who have had antibiotic(s) treatment. It is responsible for several nosocomial outbreaks especially in geriatric and long-stay wards. The symptom is mainly diarrhoea which usually starts 5-10 days (range few days to 2 months) after commencing on antibiotic therapy. It ranges from mild to severe foul smelling diarrhoea containing blood/mucous, fever, leucocytosis and abdominal pain. In the majority of patients, the illness is mild and full recovery is usual. Elderly patients may become seriously ill with dehydration. Occasionally, patients may develop a severe form of the disease called pseudomembranous colitis. Complications include pancolitis, toxic megacolon, perforation or endotoxin shock. The following are the main predisposing factors:

- elderly patients; outbreaks being more common in geriatric and long-stay wards.

- patients with underlying disease.

- patients on antibiotic therapy (in particular broad spectrum antibiotics).

- post-surgical patients.

All suspected cases should be investigated by sending faecal specimens to the microbiology laboratory for detection of *C.difficile* toxin. Usually, once the diagnosis has been confirmed, repeat specimens need not be taken unless there is a relapse following treatment because it is not uncommon for the faeces to remain positive for some time after the start of treatment even when the patients symptoms have settled. Screening and treatment of asymptomatic patient's is unnecessary.

Fortunately, most patients develop only a mild illness and stopping the antibiotic(s) together with fluid replacement to rehydrate patients usually results in rapid improvement. Sometimes, however, it is necessary to give specific therapy, ie oral metronidazole 400 mg 8 hourly for 7-10 days which should be given as first choice. If metronidazole is not effective then **oral** vancomycin 125 mg 6 hourly for 7-10 days should be prescribed.

The majority of patients improve within 2-4 days, however clinical relapse usually occurs within 1-3 weeks in 15-25% cases for which advice from the medical microbiologist should be sought. The use of opiates and antiperistaltic drugs **must** be avoided as these may cause toxic megacolon.

Patients with diarrhoea, especially if severe or accompanied by incontinence, may spread the infection to other patients. *C.difficile* has the ability to form spores which survive in the environment for months. They are highly resistant to most disinfectants and, therefore present cross-infection risk to other patients for quite a long period. The following infection control precautions should be taken:

- All Infected patients should be segregated from non-affected patients in a single room with en suite toilet facilities or cohort all symptomatic patients, using enteric isolation precautions (see 27).

- Hands can become contaminated by direct contact with patients who are colonized or infected with *C.difficile* or by contact with spores contaminating the environmental surfaces. Therefore, strict hand washing before and after patient contact remains the most effective control measure in preventing person-to-person spread of this infection.

- Staff should wear non-sterile, single-use disposable gloves and disposable plastic aprons when caring for infected patients. Hands must be washed after removing gloves.

- The patient's immediate environment and other areas where spores may accumulate, eg sluice, commodes, toilets, bedpans, sinks, floors and other soiled areas, must be cleaned thoroughly and frequently with warm water and neutral detergent. The patient's room must be cleaned daily. Separate equipment must be reserved for this purpose. Mop heads should be disposable or laundered after each use and single-use disposable cloths must be used and discarded after each use.

- Since the sensible use of antibiotics is the key to the prevention and control of *C.difficile* infection the antibiotic prescribing policy must be reviewed. Avoid the use of excessive, inappropriate and broad spectrum antibiotics (especially oral). Narrow spectrum antibiotics for a minimum duration are preferred if treatment is considered essential to treat systemic infection. Antibiotics such as aminoglycosides and some fluoroquinolones (including ciprofloxacin) appear to have little propensity to induce *C. difficile* infection, probably due to their lack of effect on the endogenous anaerobic gut bacteria.

- In the case of patient discharge or transfer the medical practitioner of the receiving health care facility should be informed about the patient's diagnosis.

Reference and further reading

Department of Health and Public Health Laboratory Service. *Clostridium difficile Infection: prevention and management* London: Department of Health, 1994.

Cartmill TDI, Panigrahi H, Worsley MA *et al.* Management and control of a large outbreak of diarrhoea due to *Clostridium difficile*. *Journal of Hospital Infection* 1994; **27**: 1-15.

Hoffman PN. *Clostridium difficile* in hospitals. *Current Opinion in Infectious Diseases* 1994; **7**: 471-474.

Tabaqchali S, Jumaa P. Diagnosis and management of *Clostridium difficile* infection. *British Medical Journal* 1995; **310**: 1375-1380.

Bartlett JG. *Clostridium difficile*: History of its role as an enteric pathogen and the current state of knowledge about the organism. *Clinical Infectious Diseases* 1994; **18** (Suppl 4): S265-272.

LEGIONNAIRES' DISEASE

Legionnaires' disease is caused by *Legionella pneumophila*. It is an acute bacterial disease characterized initially by anorexia, malaise, myalgia and headache. Within a day, there is usually a rapidly rising fever associated with chills. A nonproductive cough, abdominal pain and diarrhoea are common. Chest radiograph may show patchy or focal areas of consolidation that may progress to bilateral involvement and ultimately to respiratory failure. The case-fatality rate has been as high as 40% in hospitalized cases; it is generally higher in those with compromised immunity.

Most cases of Legionnaires Disease have occurred in a population aged between 40-70 years with males affected more commonly than females. Illness is especially common among smokers and patients with underlying medical condition, eg diabetes mellitus, chronic lung disease, renal disease, malignancy, immunocompromized and organ recipients. Outbreaks have occurred among hospitalized patients. Unrecognized infections are common. The incubation period of Legionnaires' disease is 2-10 days, most often 5-6 days.

Pontiac fever is not associated with pneumonia or death; patients recover spontaneously in 2-5 days without treatment. This clinical syndrome may represent reaction to inhaled antigen rather than bacterial invasion

In the UK, the National Surveillance Scheme for Legionnaires' Disease at the PHLS Communicable Disease Surveillance Centre has given the guidance (see reference) and the following case definition of Legionnaires' Disease:

Confirmed case: A clinical diagnosis of pneumonia with laboratory evidence of one or more of the following:

- culture of *Legionella* spp. from clinical sepcimens.
- seroconversion (a fourfold rise or greater) to 64 or more by the indirect immunofluorescent antibody test (IFAT) using *L. pneumophila* serogroup 1 yolk sac antigen.
- seroconversion (a fourfold rise or greater to 16 or more by the rapid microagglutination test (RMAT) using *L. pneumophila* serogroup 1 antigen.

Presumptive case: A clinical diagnosis of pneumonia with laboratory evidence of one or more of the following:

- a single titre of 128 or more using IFAT as above (64 or more in an adult outbreak).
- a single titre of 32 or more using RMAT as above.
- positive urine ELISA using validated reagents.
- positive direct fluorescence (DFA) on a clinical specimen using validated monoclonal antibodies.

Reservoir and source of infection for Legionnaires' Disease are domestic hot and cold water systems (showers) particularly in hospitals and hotels, air-conditioning and wet cooling system towers, evaporative condensers, humidifiers, whirlpool and natural spas, respiratory therapy devices and decorative fountains/sprinkler systems. Its main mode of spread is via the respiratory tract. Person-to-person transmission has not been documented.

The diagnosis of Legionellosis is difficult on purely clinical criteria and reliance is therefore placed on laboratory tests which include isolation of the causative organism on special media and its demonstration by direct Immunofluorescence (IF) stain of involved tissue or respiratory secretions. It can also be diagnosed by detection of antigens of *L. pneumophila* in urine by RIA or by a fourfold or greater rise in IFA titre between an acute phase serum and one drawn 3-6 weeks later.

Currently there is no vaccine against Legionellosis and since Legionella is a very widespread organism, prevention must therefore focus on reducing the risk of the organism being aerosolised. The prime aim must be to avoid creating conditions favourable for the organisms to multiply in water and be disseminated in air through droplets which are inhaled by susceptible persons leading to Legionnaires' Disease. This can be achieved by proper design and adequate maintenance of wet cooling towers and hot water systems. It is important that cooling towers should be drained when not in use. They should be mechanically cleaned to remove scale and sediment at regular intervals. Appropriate biocides should be used to prevent the growth of slime-forming organisms. Tap water should not be used in respiratory therapy devices. Maintenance of hot water system temperatures at ≥50°C may reduce the risk of transmission. Decontamination of implicated sources by chlorination and/or superheating of the water supply has been effective.

All cases of Legionnaires' Disease **must** be reported immediately to the local Consultant in Communicable Disease Control; in hospital the Infection Control Doctor must also be informed. The CCDC will investigate the contacts and source of infection and will search for additional cases due to infection from a common environmental source. Following a single confirmed nosocomial case, the CCDC and the ICD will initiate investigation from a hospital source. CCDC is also responsible for:

- Epidemic measure including search for common exposures among cases and possible environmental sources of infection.

- Convene Outbreak Control Group, if necessary, to take appropriate action, ie carry out epidemiological investigations, collection of clinical specimens for microbiology, collection of water samples etc.

- CCDC will co-ordinate the investigation and implement measures to control the outbreak.

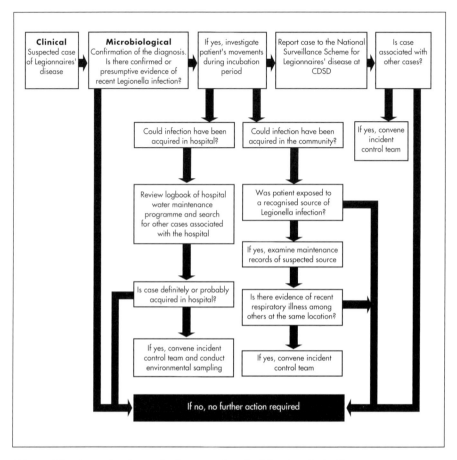

Figure 4.3 – Investigating a single case of aquired Legionaire's disease.
(Reproduced with permission from the *Communicable Disease Report* 1994;**4(10)**:R112-114).

References and further reading

Health and Safety Commission. *The prevention and control of Legionellosis (including Legionnaires' Disease). Approved Code of Practice.* London: HMSO, 1995.

Health and Safety Executive. *The control of Legionellosis including Legionnaires' Disease.* London: HMSO, 1991.

Department of Health. NHS Estates. *Health technical Memorandum 2040: The control of Legionella in health care premises - a code of practice.* London: HMSO, 1993.

British Standards Institute. *BS7592:1992 sampling for Legionellae organisms in water and related materials* London: British Standards Institute, 1992.

Joseph CA, Watson JM, Harrison TG, Bartlett CLR. Nosocomial Legionnaires' Disease in England and Wales, 1980-1992. *Epidemiology and Infection* 1994; **112:** 329-345.

Fallon RJ. How to prevent an outbreak of Legionnaires' disease. *Journal of Hospital Infection* 1994; **27:** 247-256.

Bartlett CLR, Macrae Ad, Macfarlane JT. *Legionella Infections* London: Edward Arnold, 1986.

Brundrett GW. *Legionella and Building Services* Oxford: Butterworth-Heinemann, 1992.

Health and Safety Executive. *The control of Legionellosis including Legionnaires' disease.* Health and Safety Series Booklet *HS(G)70* London: HMSO, 1991.

Saunders CJP, Joseph CA,Watson JM. Investigating a single case of Legionnaires' disease: guidance for consultants in communicable disease control. *Communicable Disease Report* 1994;**4:**R112-114.

MULTIPLY-RESISTANT GRAM-NEGATIVE BACILLI

Gram-negative bacilli include *Klebsiella, Citrobacter, Serratia, Enterobacter, Proteus* spp, *Pseudomonas aerogenosa* etc. These organisms can cause hospital-wide problems because of their ability to acquire resistance to antibiotics. Multiple antibiotic-resistant Gram-negative bacilli are more widespread in the hospital environment as a result of broad-spectrum antibiotic usage and advanced invasive techniques.

Wet environments in the hospital are the major reservoir of these organisms and may provide a common source of organisms when there is failure of standard infection control practice. They are spread between patients from health care workers and attendants by contaminated hands from the environment. The following measures are required to control these organisms:

- Compliance to hand washing procedures is essential.

- Patients in a special unit eg neonatal, intensive care, ophthalmic, neurosurgical, burns units or areas where patients are treated with immunosuppressive drugs should be isolated in single rooms with contact isolation precaution (see page 26) to prevent cross-infection to the highly susceptible patients.

- Patients should not be transferred between wards or hospital unless it is absolutely essential. If transfer is essential the Infection Control Team should be informed who will inform the receiving hospital/unit regarding the necessary infection control precautions.

- Heat treat bedpans and urinals. If a bedpan disinfector breaks down this should be repaired as an emergency. Dedicated bedpans should be used for patients with multi-resistant organisms.

- Communal equipment may act as a source for these organisms, therefore ward equipment must be stored dry, and soaking of instruments in disinfectant solution **must** be avoided. Ward equipment should be heat disinfected; disinfectant solutions are not substitute for heat disinfection.

- Insertion of urinary catheters should carried out as an aseptic procedure. Urine drainage bags must be emptied by the tap, for which single-use disposable gloves should be used and hands should be washed after theprocedure. Do not break the circuit and reconnect. A separate jug or container should be used for each patient when emptying urinary drainage bags.

- Excessive use of broad spectrum antibiotics should be discouraged. Antimicrobial prophylaxis for surgery should be restricted to a maximum of 24 hours.

VANCOMYCIN RESISTANT ENTEROCOCCI

The incidence of nosocomial colonization and infections due to *Enterococci* spp. (*E. faecalis and E. faecium*) has been rising steadily since the 1980s. At the same time, these bacteria have acquired resistance to ampicillin/amoxacillin, aminoglycosides (high level) and glycopeptides (vancomycin and teicoplanin). Patients infected with vancomycin resistant enterococci (VRE) present a challenge for physicians, as the treatment options are often limited to combining antimicrobials or experimental compounds that have unproven efficacy. The epidemiology of VRE has not been clarified, however the following patient populations are at increased risk of infection or colonization:

- treatment with previous vancomycin and/or multi-antimicrobial chemotherapy.

- critically ill patients (eg patients in ICU, oncology or transplant wards).

- severe underlying disease or immunosuppression.

- patients who have had intra-abdominal or cardio-thoracic surgery procedure and/or an indwelling urinary or central venous catheter with prolonged stay in hospital.

Enterococci can be found in the normal gastrointestinal and female genital tracts and most enterococcal infections have been attributed to endogenous sources within the individual patient. However, recent reports of outbreaks and endemic infection caused by enterococci, including VRE, have indicated that patient-to-patient transmission of the microorganisms can occur either through direct or indirect contact via hands of personnel or contaminated patient-care equipment or environmental surfaces.

Eradication of VRE from hospitals is most likely to succeed when infection or colonization is confined to a few patients on a single ward. After VRE has become endemic on a ward, or has spread to multiple wards, eradication becomes difficult and costly. Aggressive infection control measures and strict compliance by hospital personnel is required to limit nosocomial spread. The following infection control measures are recommended to prevent patient to patient transmission :

- Isolate all infected or colonized patients in a side room or cohort them with other patients.

- Dedicated instruments should be used on infected or colonized patient(s), eg stethoscope, rectal thermometers, sphygmomanometer etc. Surfaces should be cleaned and disinfected with alcohol. Adequate cleaning and disinfection of these devices must be carried out if such devices are re-used on other patients.

- Wear non-sterile disposable gloves when in contact with infected or colonized patients or their environment. Hands are subsequently disinfected with alcoholic chlorhexidine ("Hibisol").

- Environmental cleaning using hot water and detergent should be done on a regular basis.

- Transfer of patients to other high dependency units must be restricted If considered essential, seek advice from a member of the Infection Control Team.

- Screening swabs for culture from multiple body sites, ie stool or rectal swabs, perineal area, mouth, axillae, area of broken skin, (ie ulcer and wound), CSU from catheterized patients, colostomy site should be taken to identify carriers or in an outbreak situation, as advised by the Infection Control Team.

- Antibiotic policy should be reviewed in an attempt to reduce use of all broad spectrum antibiotics and use of glycopeptide.

Patients can remain colonized for a long time after discharge from hospital therefore it is important that these patients (infected or colonized) should be promptly identified and placed on isolation precautions upon re-admission to the hospital. If patients require transfer to another hospital, a member of the Infection Control Team of the receiving hospital must be informed.

References and further reading

The Hospital Infection Control Practices Advisory Committee. Recommendations for preventing the spread of vancomycin resistance. *Morbidity and Mortality Weekly Report* 1995;**44**:1-13.

Spera RV, Faber BF. Multiply-resistant *Enterococcus faecium*. The nosocomial pathogen of the 1990s. *Journal of American Medical Association* 1992;**268**:2563-2564.

Wade JJ, Uttley. Resistant enterococci - mechanisms, laboratory detection and control in the hospitals. *Journal of Clinical Pathology* 1996;**49**:700-703.

Boyce JM. Vancomycin-Resistant Enterococcus: Detection, Epidemiology, and Control Measures. *Infectious Disease Clinics of North America* 1997; **11(2)**: 367-384.

VIRAL HAEMORRHAGIC FEVERS

The Viral Haemorrhagic Fevers (VHF) are endemic in west and central Africa. Their countries of origin are – *Lassa fever:* Nigeria, Sierra Leone and Liberia; *Marburg disease:* Uganda, Kenya, Zimbabwe; *Ebola fever:* Zaire and Sudan; *Conga/Crimean fever:* former Soviet Union and east and west Africa. All have a significant mortality rate and there is no vaccine available. The incubation period of the infection is usually 7-10 days (ranging from 3-17 days). For infection control purposes, if no infection has occurred in a period of up to 21 days from exposure, a contact is usually taken to be free from infection.

A firm diagnosis is not always possible but both the clinical and the epidemiological evidence needs to be considered for any patient presenting with undiagnosed fever within 3 weeks of return from an endemic area. The most important clinical signs includes pyrexia, sore throat, rigor, nausea, vomiting and diarrhoea, headache, haemorrhage and myalgia. These symptoms should be recorded. History of adequate malarial prophylaxis must be taken. Malaria is a common confounding diagnosis and is suspected in patients who have failed to take adequate malarial prophylaxis. Risk categories have been updated as follows:

Risk categories

Minimum risk: Patients for whom the possibility of a VHF has been assessed whose history and clinical condition make the diagnosis unlikely. This category includes febrile patients who were not in known endemic or outbreak areas before they became ill, or who were in such areas but became ill more than 21 days after contact with a potential source of infection, and patients whose risk category has been revised because of their clinical condition or the results of laboratory tests. These patients can be managed with standard isolation techniques in standard facilities, and standard ambulance transport is appropriate. A thin blood film for malaria is urgent. Statutory notification is not recommended.

Moderate risk: Febrile patients who have been in an endemic area during the 21 days before they became ill but who have no other risk factors, or who have not been in an endemic area but may have been in adjacent areas and who have evidence of severe illness with organ failure and/or haemorrhage, with no current alternative diagnosis. Few patients remain in this category for more than 48 to 72 hours. These patients should be admitted either to a Department of Health designated high security infectious disease (HSID) unit or to intermediate isolation facilities and transported by a category ambulance. Malaria will be the final diagnosis in more than 95% of cases, and virological test for VHF are generally not indicated. Specimens other than the initial thin blood film for malaria, should be sent only to an HSID laboratory. The proper officer, generally the Consultant in Communicable Disease Control (CCDC), should be notified and contacts identified, but the contacts need not be placed under surveillance unless the patient is reclassified as high risk.

High risk: Febrile patients who have been in an endemic area during the three weeks before illness and have lived in or stayed in a house for more than four hours where there were febrile people known or strongly suspected to have a VHF or have cared for a febrile patient known or strongly suspected to have a VHF, or have had contact with body fluids, tissue, or a dead person or animal known to have had a VHF, or were previously classified as moderate risk, but have developed organ failure and/or haemorrhage. This category also includes febrile patients who have not been in an endemic area, but have cared for a patient or animal known or strongly suspected to have had a VHF during the three weeks before they themselves became ill. High risk patients should be admitted to an HSID unit and all specimens (except the initial malaria test) must be handled in an HSID laboratory. The CCDC should be notified. All those who had close contact with the patient after onset of illness should have their temperatures taken daily for 21 days after their last contact.

Laboratory investigation

Most laboratory tests in patients with suspected VHF are not encouraged in the initial assessment because the collection and handling of laboratory specimens is the commonest source of VHF in health care settings. General hospitals may conduct emergency tests under the guidance HSID specialist in exceptional life threatening circumstances. Laboratory procedures must include a risk assessment at each stage, including risks associated with the chosen techniques, recommendation about training and surveillance measures, waste disposal and decontamination. The two HSID laboratories for England and Wales are the PHLS Virus Reference Division, Central Public Health Laboratory, Colindale Avenue, London, (tel 0181 200 4400) and the Centre for Applied Microbiology and Research, Porton Down, Salisbury, (tel 01980 612100).

In general practice

If the General Practitioners have seen a patient at home and have suspected a diagnosis of VHF in a patients suffering from acute atypical fevers, especially with any accompanying superficial haemorrhages, in patients who have recently returned from endemic areas, they are advised not to move the patients from home and seek advice from the Consultant Physician in Infectious Diseases and should arrange to send the patients to the HSID. They should also inform the Consultant in Communicable Disease Control (CCDC) as a matter of urgency. The CCDC and the Consultant Physician in Infectious Diseases will advice the ambulance service about the danger of infection and transport the patient using a stretcher plastic film isolator.

In hospital

There is nevertheless, the possibility that such provisional diagnosis might first be made in a patient attending hospital as an out-patient eg in the Accident & Emergency department or in a patient already in a general hospital ward. The following action must be taken:

- The patient must be isolated in a single room with strict isolation precautions (see page 20) and **must not** be moved from the suspected ward or department.

- Consultant Physician in Infectious Diseases and HSID unit must be contacted for advice. Infection Control Doctor of the hospital and CCDC must be informed as a matter of urgency.

- The absolute minimum of staff may have contact with the patient, ie one doctor and one nurse. The doctor involved in making the initial diagnosis should seek advice from the Consultant Physician in Infectious Diseases. In such circumstances no other hospital medical staff should be invited to assist in confirming suspicions to minimize the risk to health care workers.

- Staff already involved with the case must not resume other professional duties and should remain, as far as possible, within the department, using a designated staff room. Instruments, dressings, documents, clothing or any other item must not be removed from the area.

The CCDC will notify the case to the following:

- Hospital Chief Executive/manager or deputy out-of-hour.

- Communicable Disease Surveillance Centre, PHLS, London.

- In consultation with the Infection Control Doctor and the Occupational Health Department arrange any necessary continuing isolation and surveillance for staff who have been in contact with the patient.

- In consultation with a member of the Infection Control Team, arrange any necessary decontamination measures of room and equipment.

- In conjunction with the relevant senior medical and nursing personnel determine if:

  - any surveillance measures are necessary in regard to other patients who may have been in contact with suspect case.

  - any restrictions are appropriate in admissions, discharge or transfers from the ward or department or any restrictions on visiting.

References and further reading

Advisory Committee on Dangerous Pathogens. *Management and control of viral haemorrhagic fever* London: The Stationary Office, 1997.

Management of patients with suspected viral haemorrhagic fever. *Morbidity and Mortality Weekly Report* (Supplement), 1988; **37:** 1–16.

RABIES

In the UK, virtually all cases of rabies have been imported from other countries. Human-to-human transmission of rabies is very rare and has been demonstrated in patients who have received infected corneal grafts. Transmission is mostly from an animal bite in countries where rabies is prevalent. Incubation period is usually 3-8 weeks, but may be as short as 9 days or as long as 7 years, depending on the severity of the wound, site of the wound in relation to the richness of the nerve supply and its distance from the brain. If the history reveals any significant exposure specialist advice must be taken .

Ideally, patients should be assessed in their own home by the Consultant Physician in Infectious Diseases. General practitioners are advised that if they are dealing with a suspected case of rabies, then they should immediately contact the Consultant Physician in Infectious Diseases who will see the patient at home. Consultant in Communicable Disease Control (CCDC) must also be informed urgently, who will advise and organize the transport of the patients to the hospital.

However, for a range of reasons, patients may be admitted to hospital before rabies is suspected. Many hospitals will have necessary facilities to undertake isolation nursing within an intensive care unit; where such facilities do not exist the patient should be admitted to a hospital in the nearest district which must be arranged in advance. The Infection Control Doctor of the hospital and CCDC must be informed as a matter of urgency.

Rabies is transmitted when infected saliva contaminates mucous membrane or an open wound. The following precautions are recommended:

- The patient should be isolated in a single room, preferably in an Intensive Care Unit. The staff must wear protective clothing including gloves, gown, goggles etc.

- Mouth-to-mouth resuscitation should not be used.

- Minimum of medical and nursing staff should be involved in the investigation and treatment.

- Staff with open lesions should not be allowed to have contact with the patient.

- Pregnant female staff should not attend the patient.

- Specimens from the patient should not be sent to routine diagnostic laboratories without prior consultation with the consultant microbiologist and/or consultant virologist.

- Equipment soiled by secretions or excretions must be destroyed or autoclaved using heat sterilization in the CSSD.

- Attendant staff and other close contacts should be offered immunization and sometimes rabies specific immunoglobulin at the advice of the CCDC, Infection Control Doctor or Consultant Physician in Infectious Diseases.

- Post-mortem examination should not be undertaken. Where such examination may be of value the indications and arrangements must be discussed with the consultant histopathologist.

In the UK, advice on pre- and post-exposure prophylaxis is available from the Communicable Disease Surveillance Centre, telephone 0181 200 6868 or the Public Health Laboratory Virus, Reference Division, telephone 0181 200 4400 and the Scottish Centre for Infection and Environmental Health, telephone 0141 946 7120.

References and further reading

Department of Health and Social Security. *Memorandum on rabies* London: HMSO, 1977.

Rabies Prevention - United States 1991. Recommendations of the Immunization Practices Advisory Committee. *Morbidity and Mortality Weekly Report* 1991;**40:**1–19.

Department of Health, Welsh Office, Scottish Office Department of Health, DHSS (N. Ireland). *Immunization against infectious disease* London: HMSO, 1996.

CREUTZFELDT-JAKOB DISEASE

Creutzfeldt-Jakob Disease (CJD) is a progressive degenerative disease of the brain which causes dementia and death, usually within 6 months of diagnosis. It is caused by unconventional transmissible agents known as prions. Most cases of CJD in the UK and elsewhere occur sporadically, but up to 15% of the cases may be familial and associated with a mutation in a gene that encodes prion protein (PrP). The incubation period of sporadic cases of CJD is unknown, but iatrogenic cases appear to have an incubation period of 2 to 15 years or more, depending on the route of inoculation.

CJD has been transmitted accidentally in human sources including growth hormones, dura mater preparation and transplantation of a corneal graft donated by an affected patient. There is no convincing evidence of case-to-case transmission of CJD nor of spread of the disease to medical, nursing or laboratory personnel who have come in contact with patients, or with nervous and other tissue derived from them.

The diagnosis can be made on clinical grounds based on the history of rapidly progressive dementia, the presence of mycolonic movements and a characteristic electroencephalogram. It can be confirmed by the histological examination of brain tissue after death.

The CJD agent is a category 2 pathogen which presents special hazards in that it survives formalin fixation, therefore all formalin-fixed specimens should be regarded as still being infective. It has also a high degree of resistance to physical and chemical procedures employed for sterilization and disinfection. Therefore all biopsy specimens, specimens of blood and CSF should be placed in the appropriate containers, enclosed in plastic bags and labelled "Danger of Infection - Take Special Care". Special care should therefore be taken to avoid accidental inoculation or other contamination while preparing the tissue for microscopy.

CJD patients should not be accepted as blood donors, and none of their tissues used for transplant purposes. In the case of corneal grafts, precautions should be taken that the member of the ophthalmic surgical team responsible for collecting the corneas should be instructed to make specific enquiries to exclude such cases. Corneas should not be taken from demented patients nor from those who die in psychiatric hospitals, nor from patients who die from obscure undiagnosed neurological diseases.

Isolation of CJD patients is unnecessary as the risk of person-to-person transmission presented by such patients in the ward is considered to be negligible. However, when procedures, ie lumbar punctures for radiological and other investigations, biopsies, dressing wounds and venepuncture/administration of injections are carried out, the health care worker should wear single-use disposable plastic apron and gloves. Disposable drapes and dressings should be used. Single-use disposable items should be used and destroyed by incineration.

For surgical procedures on CJD patients not involving brain or spinal cord, and for dental procedures, members of the operating team should wear single-use disposable protective clothing, ie fluid repellent operative gowns, gloves, masks, caps, overshoes, a disposable plastic apron under the operation gown and suitable eye protection. Only disposable drapes and dressings must be used and destroyed after use. Disposable instruments and equipment should be used wherever possible.

Where the surgical procedure involves the brain (eg cortical biopsy), spinal cord, or eye, the following additional precautions should be taken:

- the least possible number of persons should take part in the operation.

- a one-way flow of instruments should be maintained.

- when it is necessary to use instruments which are not normally regarded as disposable, these instruments must not be re-used but destroyed by incineration.

These precautions should also be observed when neurosurgical procedures are carried out on patients in whom the possibility of CJD enters into the differential diagnosis.

Post-mortem on patients with CJD should be done by a neuropathologist with access to a specialized "high risk" mortuary. However, a general histopathologist who has been asked to perform a necropsy on a case of possible or probable CJD must follow suitable infection control precautions based on guidance issued by the Health and Safety Commission and Advisory Committee on Dangerous Pathogens.

In summary, disposable equipment should not be re-used; other instruments should be re-used only if they can be subjected to the autoclaving (heat sterilization) procedures. Special care must be taken by the pathologist and the post-mortem room attendants to avoid any accidental penetration of the skin during the procedure. As few persons as possible should take part in the autopsy or be in the post-mortem room. Personal protective equipment must be worn. The bodies of patients who have died with CJD must not be used for teaching anatomy or pathology.

Great care should be taken to avoid cuts and sharps injuries, particularly from contact with sharp bony edges and during sewing up. Accidental injuries or inoculation wounds should be thoroughly washed (without scrubbing) in running water immediately, and reported to Occupational Health Department or the Accident & Emergency department according to local policy. An official record must be made of any such accident. It should be emphasised that no case of infection transmitted in this way has been recorded.

References and further reading

Advisory Committee on Dangerous Pathogens. *Precautions for work with human and animal transmissible spongiform encephalopathies*. London: HMSO, 1994.

HSS (MD) 18/92. *Surgical procedures on patients with or suspected of having, or at risk of developing, Creutzfeldt-Jakob Disease (CJD), or Gerstmann-Sträussler-Scheinker Syndrome (GSS)*. DHSS, December 1992.

Bell JE, Ironside JW. How to tackle a possible Creutzfeldt-Jakob Disease necropsy. *Journal of Clinical Pathology* 1993;**46:**193-197.

INFESTATIONS WITH ECTOPARASITES

Humans are the only reservoir for these parasites, which are usually localised to a specific site of the body.

Lice (pediculosis)

There are many different species of lice but there are only three which are clinically important from family pediculidae. They can be caught only by close contact, ie close enough for a lice to walk on to another host. Lice can found off the body on bedding, chairs, floor etc. They are either dead, injured or dying and not able to crawl on to another host. The nits are the eggs of lice which are firmly attached to hair and are difficult to remove.

Infestations with lice may result in severe itching and excoriation of the scalp or body. Secondary bacterial infection may occur due to severe itching resulting in regional lymphadenitis (especially cervical).

Head louse *(Pediculus humanus var. capitis):* This species lives on the head and eyebrow hair. The female louse lays eggs at the base of the hairs where it is warmest. Transmission to another host occurs when two heads are in direct contact allowing lice to crawl on to a new head. Lice prefer clean hair where they can move around easily. They are invariably acquired from family members or close friends who should be checked for infection. Head lice cannot be transmitted to others on clothing or linen and therefore no precautions are necessary. Patients with head lice need not be isolated, except in paediatric wards where close contact between children may transmit the lice. Outbreak, of head lice are common among children in schools and institutions everywhere.

Public or Crab louse *(Phthirus pubis):* They live on coarse body hair, usually the pubic area; they may also infect facial hair (including eye lashes), axillae and body surfaces. They are transmitted by close physical contact, frequently, but not always, by sexual contact. Children may acquire crab lice through close contact with their mother, eg axillary hair. Crab lice on clothing or bedding are not transmitted to other people and can be removed by washing clothes in hot cycle.

Body louse *(Pediculus humanus var. corporis):* Body lice are still prevalent among populations with poor personal hygiene, especially in cold climates where heavy clothing is worn and bathing is infrequent. They live in clothing, not hair and go to the body only to feed. Transmission occurs in overcrowded conditions by contact with infested clothing. They are easy to eradicate as they will die if the clothing is not worn for 3 days.

Control measures

- Carefully remove all clothing of patients with body or pubic lice and seal in a bag. As lice dislike light, clothing should be handled in bright conditions. Single use non-sterile disposable gloves and a plastic apron should be worn. In hospital, process linen as infected linen according to local policy.

- No special treatment of the environment is required as spread is by personal contact. Body lice are, however, capable of surviving for a limited time in stored clothing, but head and pubic lice rapidly die when detached from their host.

- Patients with body lice do not require specific treatment but should be bathed. Infestation with head and crab lice should be referred to the medical practitioner for appropriate treatment.

- Clothing, bedding and fomites should be treated with hot water cycle (60°C or more).

Fleas

Infestation is usually with dog, cat, or bird fleas which will bite humans in the absence of the preferred host. The human flea is rare. Fleas are able to survive for some months in the environment without feeding. Elimination of the host or treatment of pets and the use of suitable insecticides on environment surfaces and soft furnishing is therefore essential.

Control measures

- Remove all clothing and bedding. All laundry should be treated as infected linen according to the local policy.

- Clothing not suitable for washing may be treated with low temperature steam. Seek advice from the CSSD manager.

- The laundry bag must be removed immediately from the ward. In laundry, the inner hot water soluble plastic bag will allow transfer to machine without handling.

- Identify the flea, and if possible, treat or remove the host. If it is a cat flea, take steps to exclude feral cats from the site.

- Vacuum clean floors, carpets, upholstery, fabrics, etc.

- Contact your pest control officer to treat the environment, eg ducting, hard surfaces, and under fixtures, with a residual insecticide if necessary.

Scabies

Scabies is caused by *Sarcoptes scabiei*. The severe itching is caused by an allergic reaction to the presence of a small mite which burrows into the top layer of skin. Consequently, the reaction does not appear immediately, but develops between 4 to 6 weeks after infection. However, symptoms may appear earlier (1 to 4 days) if the patient has had previous exposure. Patient symptom is intense itching due to hypersensitivity.

It is transmitted from person-to-person contact only after prolonged and intimate contact. Hand-holding or patient support for long periods is probably responsible for most hospital-acquired scabies. Spread from bedding, clothing or fomites is unlikely.

"Norwegian" or "crusty" scabies occur in elderly or immunosuppressed patients, ie patients on immunosuppressive therapy, AIDS, and patients with other malignancies. This form of scabies is highly contagious because mites multiply rapidly and large numbers of the parasites are present in the exfoliating scales.

Control measures

- Refer members of the family and those in close physical contact to their general practitioner so that they can be treated if necessary.
- Treat bedding and clothing as infected linen according to the local policy.
- Protective long sleeved gowns and gloves should be worn. Prolonged contact should be avoided.
- No special environmental control measures are necessary.
- For hospitalized patients, contact isolation for 24 hours after start of effective therapy.
- Patients with "Norwegian" scabies are highly contagious and isolation precautions are recommended till the treatment is completed.

References and further reading

Lettau LA. Nosocomial transmission and infection control aspects of parasitic and ectoparasitic disease. Part III. Ectoparaistes/Summary and conclusions. *Infection Control and Hospital Epidemiology* 1991; **12:** 179-185.

Maunder J. Treatments for eradicating lice and scabies. *Prescriber* 1991; April **5:** 27-48.

Maunder J. An update of headlice. *Health Visitor* 1993; **66**(9): 317-318.

Maunder J. The scourge of scabies. *Chemist and Druggist* 1992; Jan **11:** 54-55.

Chv T. Identifying parasitic infestations. *Dermatology in practice* 1997; Jan/Feb:51-54.

PEST CONTROL

Every effort must be made to achieve a reasonable level of control or the eradication of pests. Apart from the possibility of disease transmission, food may be tainted and spoiled, fabric and building structure damaged. Pharaoh's ants have been responsible for the penetration of sterile packs and the invasion of patient's dressings, including those in use on a wound. Cockroaches can carry Gram-negative bacilli and spoil food. Hospital kitchens, boiler rooms, ducts & drains provide warmth, water, food and shelters for cockroaches, pharaoh's ants and other pest. Hospital management is responsible for ensuring the premises are free from pest.

Each health care facility should have a pest control programme. This may be contracted to an approved pest control operator/contractor. Protocols for conditions of contract and initiation to treat are published by the Department of Health. A trained pest control officer should be appointed in each hospital to monitor the contract. He or she should be informed of all sightings, follow them up and liaise with the pest control contractors to ensure that appropriate treatment is carried out. He or she should also carry regular inspections for pest infestation, preferable at night because many pest are nocturnal.

All staff members sighting a pest within the hospital or health care premises must report the incident by telephone to the nominated pest control officer, followed by a letter which should include the following information for recording in the Pest Control Record book:

- the location ie ward or department.
- the type of pest, if known.
- the date and frequency of sighting.
- the name of person reporting.

In areas such as wards, kitchens, stores and laundry, the line manager should notify the pest control officer who after investigation will establish the extent of the infestation. He or she will liaise closely with the pest control contractor and is responsible for follow-up and monitoring to ensure that the pest has been eradicated.

Control measures

- Treatment with insecticides and rodenticides alone is seldom sufficient but attention must also be paid to good hygiene and structural maintenance.
- Pests require food, warmth, moisture, harbourage, and a means of entry; hospital staff should be encouraged to keep food covered, to remove spillage and waste, and to avoid accumulations of static water.

- Buildings should be of sound structure and well maintained, drains should be covered, leaking pipework repaired and damaged surfaces made good.

- Cracks in plaster and woodwork, unsealed areas around pipework, damaged tiles, badly fitted equipment and kitchen units are all likely to provide excellent harbourage.

- Close-fitted windows and doors, fly screens and bird netting will help to exclude pests from the hospitals and other health care facilities.

References and further reading

Department of Health. *NHS Management Executive. Pest Control Management for the Health Services*. HSG(92)35 London: HMSO, 1992.

Barker LF. Pests in hospitals. *Journal of Hospital Infection* 1981; **2:** 5-9.

5

BLOOD-BORNE HEPATITIS AND HIV INFECTIONS

Blood-borne infections are those where infectious agents in a person's blood can be transmitted to another person giving rise to infection. In the health care setting all health care workers are reminded that they should always follow the routine infection control precautions (see box page 140) and safe working practices to prevent transmission of infection against blood-borne viruses (BBV).

Immunization against hepatitis B infection is an effective means of protection against hepatitis B virus but should not be used as a substitute for good clinical practice and not all those given the vaccine will necessarily respond. It will protect against hepatitis B infection but will not protect against hepatitis C, HIV and other viruses transmitted through blood-borne route. The term BBV used in these guidelines covers HIV, Hepatitis B, C and other blood-borne hepatitis viruses.

VIRAL HEPATITIS

To date, six types of viral hepatitis have been identified, ie hepatitis A, B, C, D, E and most recently hepatitis G. Hepatitis A and E are transmitted by faecal-oral route and therefore will not be discussed; hepatitis viruses B, C and G are transmitted by blood-borne route.

Hepatitis B virus

Hepatitis B virus (HBV) is a member of the Hepadnavirus family of DNA virus. The mean incubation period of acute HBV infection is 75 days but it may range from 45-180 days. After exposure to the virus, most infected individuals recover completely from the acute illness, however, unapparent infections are common, particularly among children. A small, and variable, proportion of individuals do not clear hepatitis B surface antigen (HBsAg), which is found circulating in blood

Table 5.1 – Interpretation of the common patterns of serological markers of hepatitis B virus infection.

	Hepatitis B surface		Hepatitis B core		Hepatitis B "e"	
	Antigen	Antibody	Antibody (IgG)	Antibody (IgM) (*)	Antigen	Antibody
Never infected	–	–	–			
Vaccinated	–	+	–			
Immune by natural infection	–	+ (†)	–			
Acute infection:						
Early	+ (‡)	–	–	–	+/–	
Late	+	–	+	+++	+	
Carrier(§):						
High infectivity	+	–	+	+/–	+	–
Low infectivity	+	–	+	–	–	+

(*) Tests for IgM are usually strongly reactive during acute infection; weaker reactivity may also be present in carriers, particularly if they are also positive for e antigen.

(†) Not detectable in 10-15% of those who have had hepatitis B in the past; core antibody may be the only marker detectable.

(‡) The first marker to become detectable during acute infection, and before any symptoms.

(§) Someone with detectable surface antigen more than six months after acute hepatitis B or first detection of antigen.

Reproduced with permission from Gilson RJC. Hepatitis B and admission to medical school. *BMJ* 1996; **313:** 830-831.

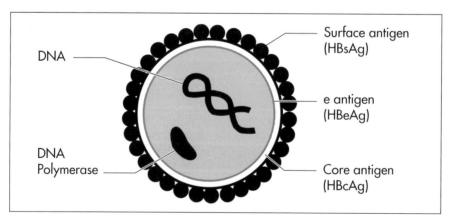

Figure 5.1 – Structure of hepatitis B virus.

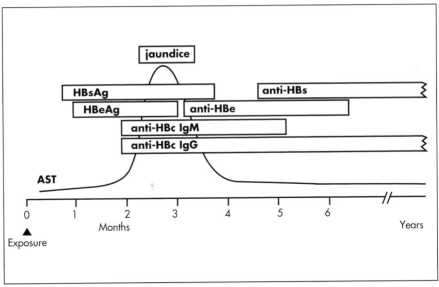

Figure 5.2 – Sequence of serological results following acute uncomplicated hepatitis. (HBsAg: hepatitis B surface antigen; Anti-HBs: antibody to hepatitis B surface antigen; HBeAg: hepatitis B e antigen; Anti-HBe: antibody to hepatitis B e antigen; Anti-HBc: antibody to core antigen; AST: asparate aminotranferase).

(Reproduced with permission from Greenough A. *et al.* In: *Congenital perinatal and neonatal infections*, 1992:89).

during the latter part of the incubation period and in the acute phase of HBV. They become carriers, (ie individuals who shed HBsAg into circulation for more than 6 months) following acute infection. Some of these develop chronic hepatitis, cirrhosis or hepatocellular carcinoma. The likelihood of a patient developing chronic hepatitis is inversely related to age at the time of infection. Chronic infection occurs in at least 90% of cases following neonatal infection, 25% of children aged 1-10 years and 5% or less in adults. Of these, 5-10% have persistent e antigenaemia (HBeAg+ve) which correlates with a high level of viral replication and heightened infectivity. These are defined as "high risk" carriers. A patient who is in the early prodromal or acute phase of hepatitis B should also be considered a high risk patient or carrier. Most carriers, however, can be classified as "low risk" with regard to transmission of infection. However, carriers of hepatitis B virus who are negative for e antigen are occasionally the source of infection. These carriers have been associated with the presence of condon mutation which stops the synthesis of e antigen but still allows production of infectious virus.

Hepatitis C virus

Hepatitis C (HCV) belongs to the flaviviridae family. Incubation periods range from 20 days to 13 weeks. The acute phase of HCV infection is usually asymptomatic or mild and patients are often unaware of the infection. Most patients will complain of fatigue but a few have a history of acute hepatitis or jaundice. If it proceeds to chronic disease, progression is usually indolent and the most common complaint is fatigue. Up to 80% of people who are anti-HCV positive may continue to carry the virus which may cause slow ongoing liver damage. It is thought that 10-20% of individuals with chronic hepatitis will go on to develop cirrhosis over 20-40 years and an unknown number of those with cirrhosis go on to develop liver cancer.

There are still no tests for detection of antigens against HCV in serum and therefore the infection is usually diagnosed by detecting antibodies against hepatitis C virus. However, detection of antibodies to HCV alone does not distinguish between individuals who have been previously exposed to the virus and those who continue to have viraemia. A Polymerase Chain Reaction (PCR) test detects small amounts of viral genetic RNA, and indicates if there is circulating virus.

Hepatitis D virus

Hepatitis D virus (HDV), previously known as the "delta agent", is a defective virus which requires the presence and the helper activity of HBV to allow it to replicate. HDV virus can be co-transmitted with hepatitis B infection or can superinfect chronic hepatitis B virus carriers. Mean incubation period is 35 days and the transmission is mainly through parenteral routes. Hepatitis caused by HDV is usually severe and individuals with double infection, HBV and HDV, usually develop rapidly progressive disease and cirrhosis at an earlier age than those with HBV infection alone.

Hepatitis G virus

The term "GB" derives from the initials of a Chicago surgeon who contracted acute hepatitis in the 1960s. So far 3 viruses have been recognised; GBV-A, GBV-B have been isolated from marmosets and a GBV-C virus has been found in samples of human sera. Hepatitis GBV-C has now been known as Hepatitis G virus (HGV); a newly discovered flavivirus. The association of the virus with liver damage is illustrated by raised in alanine aminotransferase (ALT) activities and detectable HGV RNA in a number of patients. However, between 40 and 90% of viraemic subjects have normal ALT. In a significant proportion of patients there is co-infection with HBV or HCV, or both. It has been suggested that HGV infects the human reticulo-endothelial system, ie lymphocytes or macrophages.

It can also be transmitted by blood transfusion although its role in perinatal or sexual transmission is currently unknown. More research into its epidemiology and the pathological effects is needed to understand this virus fully. The diagnosis of HGV in the clinical setting relies on the detection of RNA by PCR on blood sample.

HIV INFECTION

Human Immunodeficiency Virus (HIV) is a member of the retrovirus family and responsible for HIV infections and cases of Acquired Immunodeficiency Syndrome (AIDS). It was first isolated in 1983. HIV 2, isolated in 1986, has been distinguished from HIV 1 and is a distinct variant, prevalent in certain West African countries. The two varieties of HIV present similar hazards and cause similar illnesses, except that there is some evidence that progression of disease is slower in a person infected with HIV 2. The term HIV is used in these guidelines cover both types of virus.

Clinical features

After exposure to HIV virus, most individuals develop antibody within 3 months. During the seroconversion period (ie, time period between exposure to HIV and development of antibodies) there may be a self-limiting illness resembling glandular fever (infectious mononucleosis), lymphadenopathy and rash. After a long period, some infected individuals develop a long-lasting generalized

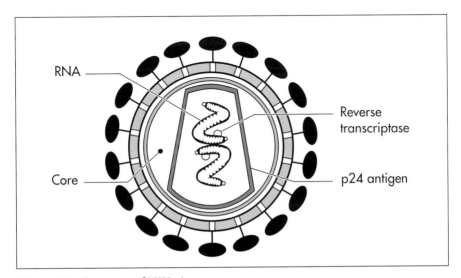

Figure 5.3 – Structure of HIV virus.

enlargement of the lymph glands. Non-specific illness (including fever, night sweats and lymphadenopathy) are associated with progressive immune dysfunction and when AIDS develops fully it is characterised by the appearance of opportunistic infections and tumours. Patients vary in their level of viraemia. Rapid progressors tend to have persistently high viral load whereas slow or non progressors have low viral load.

Infection with a yeast, *Candida* spp., may cause persistent and severe thrush in the mouth and gullet and there may be reactivation of common latent herpes viruses. Invasion of the lungs by *Pneumocystis carinii*, a microorganism normally of low virulence, often gives rise to a pneumonitis with shortness of breath and diffuse shadowing may be seen on a chest x-ray. Some individuals may be infected with *Mycobacterium* spp. ie *M.tuberculosis, M.avium-intracellulare* etc. Many other infections may supervene caused by bacteria, such as *Salmonellae*, viruses including *Cytomegalovirus* and hepatitis B and protozoa such as *Toxoplasma* in the brain or *Giardia* or *Cryptosporidium* in the bowel. Some patients develop Kaposi's sarcoma, an unusual tumour on the skin. This appears as characteristic discrete purple patches, often affecting the extremities, although internal organs may also be involved. Still others develop lymphoma, often in the brain.

Testing for HIV antibody

The diagnosis of HIV infection is confirmed by the demonstration of serum antibodies to the virus. A 5-10 ml clotted sample is required for HIV antibody testing. Laboratories carrying out the test will assume that the clinician requesting

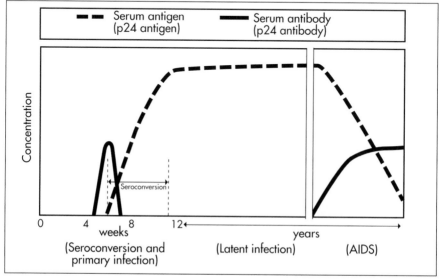

Figure 5.4 – Antigen and antibody response in HIV infection.

the investigation has obtained the necessary consent from the patient. In most virus infections, specific antibodies are usually detectable in the blood within a few weeks of infection. In the case of HIV, however, the seroconversion or *'window period'*, (ie the time between exposure to HIV infection and the first detectable sign of antibody in blood), is usually between 6 to 12 weeks but may last several months in some cases. During this *'window period'*, the HIV antibody test will be negative, therefore a negative test is not an absolute exclusion of HIV infection because the person during the period of seroconversion is still potentially infectious. Therefore, it is important that patients whose behaviour is considered to be in high risk groups should be treated with blood and body fluids infection control precautions (see page 28). After infection the virus persists in the body for life and a patient who is HIV antibody positive must therefore be considered to be permanently infectious.

Consent and counselling

In the clinical setting HIV testing can only be performed with the patient's *informed consent* and individuals should have information about HIV transmission, the significance of a positive or a negative result and be able to discuss their particular needs and concerns. All individuals requiring an HIV test should be offered appropriate discussion prior to testing. The discussion should address the specific needs of the individual requiring a test and the different clinical situations in which the HIV test is provided. The discussion about HIV and HIV testing should be part of the main stream medical care and can be carried out by any health care worker after appropriate training. However, specialist counsellors may be required if the circumstances of the individual attending for HIV testing are complex and extensive discussion would be required. Details on pre-test discussion on HIV testing is outlined in the Department of Health document (see references). Patient confidentiality is of paramount importance and they have the same rights to confidentiality as any other patient.

ROUTES OF TRANSMISSION

Blood-borne viruses are transmitted through entry of blood or high risk body fluids containing virus in to individuals and may occur by:

1. Unprotected penetrative sexual intercourse with an infected person (between men or between a man and a woman).

2. Skin puncture by blood contaminated with sharps objects, ie
   - sharing used needles and syringes among intravenous drug users.
   - receipt of tattoos, earpiercing, acupuncture, dental treatment, electrolysis etc.
   - inoculation injury to health care worker from an infected individual.

3. Child birth from an infected mother to her baby (intrauterine and peripartum)or through breast feeding.

4. Via infected blood transfusion, blood products, donations of semen, skin grafts and organ transplants from someone who is infected.

It can also be transmitted through contamination of open wounds and skin lesions, eg eczema, splashing the mucous membrane of the eye, nose or mouth and through human bites when blood is drawn.

Blood is not the only concern, as various other high risk body fluids, ie cerebrospinal, peritoneal, pleural, pericardial, amniotic, synovial fluid, semen, vaginal secretions and any other body fluids containing visible blood, and all tissues, organs and parts of bodies which are unfixed, are also hazardous. Exposure to low risk body fluids such as urine, faeces, nasal secretions, tears, saliva, sputum and vomitus present a minimal risk of blood-borne virus infection unless contaminated with blood; although they may be hazardous for other reasons as they may contain other pathogenic microorganisms. When blood is mentioned, it should be taken to include the high risk body fluids unless otherwise stated.

OCCUPATIONAL RISKS TO THE HEALTH CARE WORKER

In the health care setting, the risk of acquiring blood-borne infection is proportional to the prevalence of infection in the population served and the chance of inoculation accidents occurring during procedures. The risk of infection following percutaneous exposure to the blood from an infectious source from hepatitis B patients is estimated to be between 5 to 30 %. The risk of hepatitis C infection after percutaneous exposure to a known infected source appears to be intermediate between the risk of HBV and HIV, ie between 3-10%. Estimated risk of infection following percutaneous exposure to infected blood from an infected HIV individual is in the range of 0.2-0.5%. All health care workers must report all inoculation injuries to the Occupational Health or Accident and Emergency Department, according to the local policy.

RESPONSIBILITY OF HEALTH CARE WORKERS TO THEIR PATIENTS

Transmission of hepatitis B, C and HIV from infected health care workers to patients has been documented. Therefore, all health care workers are reminded that they have an overriding ethical duty to protect the health and safety of their patients. They are strongly advised to follow routine infection control precautions (see box on page 139) scrupulously and adopt safer working practices to prevent transmission of blood-borne viral infections to their patients.

ROUTINE INFECTION CONTROL MEASURES

(All health care workers should follow these guidelines at all times irrespective of the infectious status of the patients)

- Wash hands regularly between procedures, patients, after contact with blood or body fluids and after removing gloves.

- Cover cuts, abrasion and puncture wounds with waterproof dressings and/or gloves.*

- Health care workers with large areas of broken skin must avoid invasive procedures.

- Avoid contamination of clothes by use of appropriate protective clothing, ie impermeable gown, plastic apron.

- Wear visor or goggles/safety spectacles and a mask to protect eyes, mouth and nose if there is a risk of splashes of blood or body fluids.

- Wear rubber boots or plastic disposable overshoes when the floor or ground is likely to be contaminated.

- Avoid sharps usage wherever possible. If used then institute safe procedures for handling and disposal of needles and other sharps into an approved sharps bin. The sharps container must be closed securely when three-quarters full and disposed of by incineration.

- Used needles must not be resheathed unless there is a safe means available for doing so.

- Institute approved procedures for the sterilization and disinfection of instruments and equipment.

- Surface contamination by blood, body fluids, secretion and excretion should be decontaminated and cleaned promptly using a safe method.

- Follow a safe technique for disposal of all clinical waste according to local policy.

---

*Staff with larger wounds, eczema or other skin conditions which cannot be adequately protected by plastic gloves or impermeable dressings should be referred to the consultant in the Occupational Health Department for advice and guidance.

Those who are, or have reason to believe that they may have been exposed to these infections in whatever circumstances, must inform the Medical Director of the hospital and seek medical advice from the consultant in Occupational Health Department. They ***must not*** perform ***exposure prone*** invasive procedures (see below). The consultant in occupational medicine will advise the health care worker on their work which may need to be modified or restricted to protect patients. The Medical Director of the hospital will notify the Director of Public Health who will decide if patients need to be informed. It is extremely important that the infected health care workers receive the same rights of confidentiality as any patient seeking or receiving medical care. All matters arising from and relating to the employment of infected health care workers will be co-ordinated by the consultant in occupational health medicine in strict confidence. Advice on health care workers who are infected with blood-borne viruses is available from the UK Advisory Panel set up under the aegis of the UK Health Department, c/o Secretariat, Room 727, Wellington House, 133-155 Waterloo Road, London, SE1 8UG. Telephone 0171-972 4349 (Administrative Secretariat) or 071-972 4378 (Medical Secretariat).

All health care workers (including locum staff) who perform exposure prone procedures should be vaccinated against hepatitis B virus and their serological response checked subsequently. Any health care worker who performs exposure prone procedures and who has not yet been immunized should be tested for evidence of current infection, that is presence of hepatitis B surface antigen, as soon as possible. This may mean testing before immunization has been completed. Blood specimens for testing health care workers who perform exposure prone procedures should be collected directly by a member of the occupational health service or a person commissioned by the service.

Provided routine infection control measures are followed scrupulously the circumstances in which the blood-borne infection could be transmitted from the health care worker to a patient are restricted to ***exposure prone procedures*** which ***must not be performed by a health care worker who is either HIV or hepatitis B e antigen (HBeAg) positive.*** Health care workers who have antibodies against HCV (anti-HCV) should seek advice from the consultant in their local occupational health department.

The Department of Health has defined ***exposure prone procedures*** as those where there is a risk that injury to the worker may result in the exposure of patients's open tissues to the blood of the worker. These procedures include those where the worker's gloved hands may be in contact with sharps instruments, needle tips or sharp tissues (spicules of bone or teeth) inside a patient's open body cavity, wound or confined anatomical space where the hands or fingertips may not be completely visible at all times.

Procedures where the hands and fingertips of the worker are visible and outside the patient's body at all times, and internal examinations or procedures that do not require the use of sharp instruments, are not considered to be exposure prone, provided routine infection control precautions are adhered to at all times. Examples of such procedures include the taking of blood, setting up and maintaining IV lines, minor surface suturing and the incision of abscesses or uncomplicated endoscopies. However, the final decision about the type of work that may be taken on by an infective health care worker must be decided by the consultant in Occupational Health Department on an individual basis taking into account the specific working practices and the environment of the worker concerned.

Normal vaginal delivery in itself is not an exposure prone procedure. When undertaking a vaginal delivery an infected health care worker ***must not*** perform procedures involving the use of sharps, instruments such as infiltrating local anaesthetics or suturing of a tear or episiotomy, since fingertips may not be visible at all times and the risk of injury to the worker is greater. Neither can they perform an instrumental delivery requiring forceps or suction if infiltration of local anaesthetic or internal suturing is required. In practice this means an infected health care worker may only undertake a vaginal delivery if it is certain that a second midwife or doctor may also be present who is able to undertake all such operative interventions as might arise during the course of delivery.

INFECTION CONTROL PRECAUTIONS

Infection control precautions for patients with known or suspected to be infected with blood-borne virus should follow the isolation precautions outlined in "Blood and body fluid isolation precautions" (see page28).

In a household setting, contacts of people infected with BBV should keep their open cuts and wounds covered carefully with waterproof dressings and avoid sharing razors and toothbrushes; blood spillage should be cleaned with household bleach (diluted 1:10).

Surgical procedure

In addition to the routine infection control precautions outlined in this chapter, if the patient require surgical operation the following precautions are recommended.

- The consultant in charge of the patient is responsible for seeing that all members of the team know of the infection hazards and appropriate measures to be taken. In these circumstances the team should be limited to essential members of trained staff only. It may help theatre decontamination if such cases are last on the list, but this is not essential.

- Unnecessary equipment should be removed from the theatre in order to reduce the amount of decontamination required after the operation. Disposable drapes should be used and the mattress should be protected by a plastic sheet.

- Disposable equipment should be used wherever possible. If any item of equipment is not disposable it must be decontaminated by the CSSD. Special equipment reserved for these patients are not essential.

- Depilatory creams should be used for essential hair removal.

- All staff in the theatre should wear a disposable plastic apron under their gowns. A water-impermeable gown should be worn if gross contamination with blood or body fluids is likely. Where waterproof aprons are worn for procedures in which there is likely to be considerable dissemination of blood, it is essential that the aprons are of sufficient length to overlap with protective footwear. This is especially important for procedures carried out in the lithotomy position, since it is common for blood accumulating in the worker's lap to be channelled down into the boots.

- The surgical team should wear a mask and two pairs of gloves and skin lesions must be covered with waterproof dressings. Spectacles or goggles should be worn by those taking part in the operation to avoid conjunctival contamination or splashing.

- Fenestrated footwear must never be worn in situations where sharps are handled. For tasks involving likely dissemination of blood it is recommended that wellington boots or calf length plastic boots are worn rather than shoes or clogs. Contaminated footwear must be adequately decontaminated after use with appropriate precautions for those undertaking it.

- Variations in operative technique, such as a non-touch approach, the avoidance of passing sharp instruments from nurse to surgeon and vice versa, and new techniques of cutting (as with lasers) or of wound closure that obviate the use of sharp instruments and lessen the risk of inoculation are recommended.

- Blood should be cleaned off the patient's skin as far as possible at the end of the operation, and a wound dressing used that will contain exudate within an impervious outer covering.

- If drainage is considered necessary, closed rather than open wound drainage is recommended.

- Used needles must not be resheathed. Needles, syringes and disposable sharp instruments must be discarded into approved sharps boxes. The sharps container must be closed securely when three-quarters full.

- Surgical instruments and other tools used in operations should be put in a robust puncture-resistant container, labelled "Danger of Infection" and returned to the CSSD.

- Used linen and theatre clothing should be placed in a water soluble bag which is then placed in a second red plastic bag and marked as infected linen.

- Theatre cleaning should be carried out with a freshly prepared hypochlorite (1,000 ppm av Cl_2) solution. Walls and other surfaces do not require cleaning unless contaminated with blood. Large volumes of fluid should be used for cleaning and gloves and a plastic apron should be worn by the operator. Thorough rinsing is necessary after a hypochlorite application to minimise damage to surfaces. The theatre can be used for the next patient immediately after cleaning and drying.

- The nurse handling the patient in the recovery room should wear gloves and a plastic apron.

- Spillage of blood and body fluids should immediately be disinfected and cleaned (see page 70).

- Tissues sent to the histopathology laboratory should be put in a suitable volume of fixative solution and material must be transported in secure containers with a "Danger of infection" label.

Maternity department

- The same precautions for a known or suspected patient are necessary for maternal or caesarian section as described under surgical operation.

- The placenta should be placed inside an approved robust container and sent for incineration according to the local policy.

- The labour room may be used provided it is adequately cleaned with a freshly prepared hypochlorite (1,000 ppm av Cl_2) solution after use.

- Although the risk of transmission of infection to other patients is small it is advisable to provide the mother and child with a single room post-natally.

- Mothers with HIV/AIDS should be advised not to breast feed their baby. If the mother is infected with other blood-borne viruses, seek advice from medical microbiologist/virologist.

Protection of newborn against HBV

Those providing antenatal care will need to take steps to identify infected mothers during pregnancy and make arrangements to ensure that babies born to these mothers receive a complete course of immunisation against hepatitis B infection.

This is best done by screening women early in pregnancy. Where this has not been done it should be possible to detect carrier mothers at the time of delivery.

Specific hepatitis B Immunoglobulin (HBIG) is available for passive protection while hepatitis B vaccine confers active immunity and they are normally used in combination. Babies born to mothers who are HBeAg positive, who are HBsAg positive without e markers or where e marker status has not been determined, or who have had acute hepatitis during pregnancy, should receive specific HBIG as well as active immunisation.

The new born should be given HBIG which is available in 2 ml ampoules containing 200 IU and should be given as soon as possible after birth. If the administration of HBIG is delayed for more than 48 hours seek advice from the consultant medical microbiologist/virologist. If the immunisation with the vaccine is combined with simultaneous administration of HBIG, the injection *must* be given at a different site.

The first dose of vaccine should be given at birth or as soon as possible thereafter. HBIG should be given at a contralateral site at the same time; arrangements for the supply of HBIG should be made well in advance. Currently licensed products within the UK contain different concentrations of antigen per ml. The paediatric dose for age 0–12 years is 10 mcg (0.5 ml) of Engerix B (SmithKline Beecham) and the dose for age 0–10 years is 5 mcg (0.5 ml) of the H–B–VaxII (Pasteur Merieux MSD). The complete course of Hepatitis B immunisation regimen consists of a three-dose series of vaccine, with the first dose at the time of birth, the second dose one month later and the third dose at six months after the first dose. The vaccine should normally be given intramuscularly and the anterolateral thigh is the preferred site in infants.

Procedure after death

If a person known or suspected to be infected with a blood-borne virus dies either in hospital or elsewhere it is the duty of those with knowledge of the case to ensure that those who need to handle the body, including funeral personnel, post-mortem room and mortuary staff are aware that there is a potential risk of blood-borne viral infection. Making known a known or suspected hazard to those concerned is a statutory duty under the Health and Safety at Work Act. The discreet use of simple "Danger of infection" labelling is appropriate and is attached in such a way that it can be read through cadaver bag.

The body should be placed in a disposable body bag; absorbent material may be needed when there is a leakage from, eg surgical incisions or wound. When relatives or others wish to view the body the face may be revealed but physical contact should be discouraged as far as practicable. Where this is insisted upon, information should be given of the risk of infection. The bodies of children of mothers with BBV infections should be treated as infected.

Patients known or suspected to be infected with BBV should not be embalmed. Embalming carries a significant risk for the operator as sharp instruments need to be used and a substantial quantity of the blood is drawn.

The principles of safe practice for the mortuary must be adhered to irrespective of the infective state of the body. A full post-mortem should not be done merely to confirm the cause of death. If a post-mortem examination is necessary on such patients then this must be discussed by the physician-in-charge of the patient and with the consultant histopathologist. When post-mortem is carried out on such patients all those concerned must be suitably informed and trained in safe procedures. They must follow local written protocol based on guidance issued by the Health and Safety Advisory Committee (HSAC), Advisory Committee on Dangerous Pathogens (ACDP) and other bodies (see references).

References and further reading

Advisory Committee on Dangerous Pathogens. *Protection against blood-borne infections in the workplace: HIV and hepatitis*. London: HMSO, 1995.

Department of Health. *Guidelines for pre-test discussion on HIV testing*. London: Department of Health, 1996.

UK Health Departments. *AIDS/HIV-infected health care worker: guidance on the management of infected health care workers*. London: Department of Health, 1994.

UK Health Departments. *Protecting health care workers and patients from hepatitis B.* London: Department of Health, 1993.

NHS Executive. Addendum to HSG(93)40: *Protecting health care workers and patients from hepatitis B*. EL(96)77. September 1996.

UK Health Departments. *AIDS-HIV infected health care workers: Practical guidance on notifying patients*. London: Department of Health, 1993.

UK Health Departments. *Guidance for clinical health care workers: Protection against infection with HIV and Hepatitis viruses*. Recommendations of the Expert Advisory Group on AIDS. London: HMSO, 1990 (under revision).

Working Group of Royal College of Pathologists. *HIV infection: Hazards of transmission to patients and health care workers during invasive procedures*. London: The Royal College of Pathologists, 1992.

Report of a working group of the Royal College of Pathologists. *HIV and the practice of pathology*. London: The Royal College of Pathologists, 1995.

Report of joint working party of the Hospital Infection Society and the Surgical Infection Study Group. Risks to surgeons and patients from HIV and Hepatitis:

Guidelines on precautions and management of exposure to blood or body fluids. *British Medical Journal* 1992; **305:** 1337-1343.

Hospital Infection Society Working Party Report. Acquired Immune Deficiency Syndrome. *Journal of Hospital Infection* 1990; **15:** 7-34.

Association of Anaesthetists of Great Britain and Ireland. *A report received by Council of the Association of Anaesthetists on Blood-borne Viruses and Anaesthesia.* London: Association of Anaesthetists of Great Britain and Ireland, 1996.

Royal College of Obstetricians and Gynaecologists. *HIV infection in maternity care and gynaecology.* London: The Royal College of Obstetricians and Gynaecologists, 1990.

British Orthopaedic Association. *Guidelines for the prevention of cross-infection between patients and staff in orthopaedic operating theatres with special reference to HIV and blood-borne Hepatitis viruses.* London: British Orthopaedic Association, 1992.

Health and Safety Commission. *Safe working and the prevention of infection in clinical laboratories.* London: HMSO, 1991.

Health and Safety Commission. *Safe working and the prevention of infection in the mortuary and post-mortem room.* London: HMSO, 1991.

The Royal Institute of Public Health and Hygiene. *A Handbook of Mortuary Practice and Safety for Anatomical Pathology Technicians.* London: The Royal Institute of Public Health and Hygiene, 1994.

Healing TD, Hoffman PN, Young SEJ. The infection hazards of human cadavers. *Communicable Disease Report* 1995;**5:**R61-R68.

BMA. *A Code of Practice; The Safe Use and Disposal of Sharps.* London: British Medical Association, 1992.

HA (1/92): *Decontamination of equipment, linen or other surfaces contaminated with Hepatitis B and/or Human Immunodeficiency Viruses.* DHSS, 1992.

BMA Board of Science and Education. *A guide to hepatitis C.* London: British Medical Association, 1996.

NHS Executive. *Guidance on the microbiological safety of human tissues and organs used in transplantation.* London: Department of Health, 1996.

Department of Health Welsh Office, Scottish Office Department of Health, DHSS (NI). *Immunization against Infectious Disease.* London: HMSO, 1996.

Rhodes RS, Bell DM, eds. Prevention of transmission of blood-borne pathogen. *The Surgical Clinics of North America* 1995; **75:** 1047-1217.

Zuckerman JN, Zuckerman AJ. Hepatitis - how far down the alphabet? *Journal of Clinical Pathology* 1997; **50:** 1-2.

6

PREVENTION OF INFECTIONS IN HEALTH CARE WORKERS

The prevention of infection in health care settings requires that health care workers should use appropriate infection control precautions. All health care workers should be immunized against all vaccine preventable diseases. Transmissible infections in health care workers must be identified quickly so that they can be excluded from the work place or from direct patient contact until they are no longer infectious. The role and responsibilities of the Occupation Health Department described below are mainly concerned with the risk of infection and are only a part of their work.

- Primary health screening of all staff by questionnaire and/or medical examination.

- Keeping accurate and up-to-date records of all members of staff with infection.

- Immunization and vaccination of all existing staff at the required time interval.

- Training of all grades of staff in personal hygiene with special precautions for those particularly at risk of infection.

- Examination of staff returning to work after absence due to diarrhoea or sepsis, to ensure that the infection has cleared and to give advice to carrier.

- Determining staff contacts of the infectious disease, checking immunity and follow up if necessary. Arranging tests and possibly treatment for the staff with sepsis of hospital origin who are carriers of pathogens which may be harmful to the patients.

- Keeping records of all inoculation injuries, arranging prophylaxis following inoculation injuries and counselling of staff at risk of infection when necessary.

- Survey potential infective and toxic hazards (eg chemical disinfectant) to staff in health care facilities as outlined in the COSHH regulations.

It is important that the Occupational Health Department should liaise closely with the Infection Control Team. MRSA carriage among staff members must be notified to the Infection Control Team. Staff must not work if the have acute or chronic diarrhoeal disease or febrile respiratory illness. Catering staff need to be carefully questioned about gasterointestional infection, history of enteric fever, skin condition, recurrent sepsis and tuberculosis.

Staff who are or have reason to believe that they may have been exposed to blood-borne hepatitis (B&C) or HIV infection *must* declare this and discuss it in complete confidence with the Consultant in Occupational Health Medicine, either at the initial screening when he or she first becomes aware of their infection. The Department of Health has produced guidance on this issue. In general, such staff may require a work assessment and must avoid exposure-prone procedures (see page 140).

Staff refusing immunizations may be prohibited from working in certain areas and their work should be revived by the Consultant in Occupational Health Medicine. Any staff who are found to have made a false declaration about their previous health record may be disciplined.

PRE-EMPLOYMENT HEALTH SCREENING

The primary aim of occupational health screening is to prevent disease in the individual but a second and no less important function is to prevent transmission of infectious agents to patients. It is important that all newly employed staff in the health care setting must attend the Occupational Health Department on their first day of employment. The screening process include assessment by a health questionnaire completed by the employee, covering questions related to general health, history of infections diseases and immunization status. In addition, the presence of skin disorders such as eczema, and a history of an underlying immunosuppressive disorder might require a reassessment of the staff member's work practices. The employee must be given assurance of the complete confidentiality of the health questioning and their occupational health record.

It is the responsibility of the staff member's manager to ensure that the individual attends the Occupational Health Department and receives training in health and safety appropriate to the work to be undertaken. All new staff should be made aware of their responsibilities as an employee under the Health & Safety at Work Act, COSHH regulations and other guidelines. They should be trained in the handling of blood and body fluids, chemical agents, eg disinfectants and should be aware of local policies and procedures on infection control including waste disposal, dealing with contaminated sharps etc. They must be told to report any accidents or illness to their manager and, if appropriate, to the Occupational Health Department. All health care workers should also be provided with adequate protective materials when appropriate. Health care facilities have a responsibility to ensure that all reasonably practicable steps are taken to ensure that the risk of infection from health workers is minimised.

Agencies which provide temporary staff for the hospital should be informed of the staff screening policy and, wherever possible, only those agencies with an effective screening programme should be used.

PROTECTION AGAINST TUBERCULOSIS

All staff in regular contact with patients, and especially those working in chest medicine or investigation units, thoracic surgery units, infectious disease wards, laboratory staff working in microbiology, pathology and post-mortem rooms staff are at potential risk of contracting tuberculosis. All staff, including agency staff and locum, should be screened and offered protection with BCG vaccine pre-employment as outlined in the British Thoracic Study guidelines. Provider units which have contracts with agencies should specify that the agency only supplies staff who meet this requirement.

It is important that all prospective staff should undergo pre-employment health screening. Enquiry about symptoms suggestive of tuberculosis should form part of the pre-employment health questionnaire which should be checked by the Occupational Health Department. The results of Heaf testing and BCG vaccination should be obtained when feasible.

A Heaf test should be carried out on those prospective employees who do not have a definite BCG scar. It is not necessary to perform a Heaf test routinely on those individuals who have an identified scar.

Clinical examination, tuberculin skin testing and chest radiography must be considered by the occupational health physician when symptoms or history are suggestive of tuberculosis. If the chest x-ray is abnormal, with features requiring further investigation, referral to a respiratory physician should be arranged. If clinical investigations reveal no evidence of tuberculosis, the health care worker should be managed as for asymptomatic individuals.

A negative or grade 1 Heaf test in the absence of a definite BCG scar is an indication for BCG vaccination. Those without a satisfactory reaction require a further tuberculin test and, if this is negative, a second vaccination. Physicians may prefer to repeat the Heaf test in older persons to detect a boosted reaction and avoid unnecessary BCG vaccination.

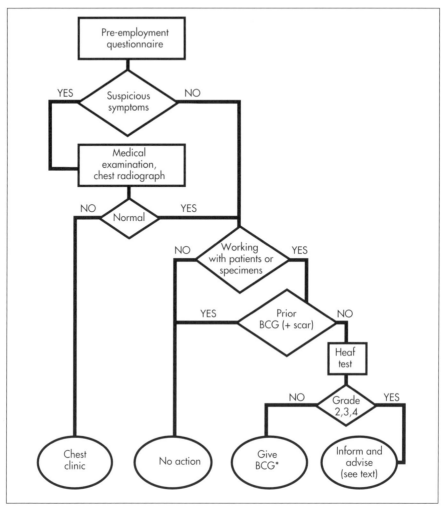

Figure 6.1 – Guidelines for Occupational Health Department for protection of health care workers against tuberculosis. *Some units may prefer to repeat the Heaf test in older persons to detect a boosted reaction and avoid unnecessary BCG vaccination.

(Reproduced with permission from the Joint Tuberculosis Committee of the British Thoracic Society. *Thorax* 1994; **49:** 1193-1200.)

Some UK workers and visiting workers from other countries where BCG is not used may not wish to receive the BCG immunisation. Individuals who have come from or have worked in high prevalence countries should undergo screening. Those without a definite BCG scar should have Heaf testing and those with a positive response (grades 2-4) should undergo clinical examination and chest x-ray. Those with strongly positive Heaf tests (grade 3 or 4) and /or relevant clinical findings should be referred to a respiratory physician for further management.

Asymptomatic individuals who have no BCG scar and on Heaf testing have a grade 2, 3 or 4 result should be advised that they have encountered *M.tuberculosis* in the past and do not require BCG vaccination. Careful enquiry must be made to ensure that they are truly asymptomatic and they must be advised of the relevant symptoms and the need to report these. A routine chest x-ray is not required.

Arrangements need to be in place so that all staff are aware that if they believe they may be immunocompromised they are advised not to receive BCG and not to work directly with patients with pulmonary tuberculosis.

Consideration should be given to the need for education of health care workers, including reminders of the symptoms of tuberculosis (especially for those at greater exposure) so that they can seek advice early if problems arise.

If prospective employees refuse consent to a Heaf test, chest x-ray or BCG, then the Occupational Health Department may decline to pass the individual fit for work. Alternatively they may place restrictions on where the individual may be deployed.

Post-exposure management: Following exposure of staff to a patient with open pulmonary (positive sputum smear for AAFB) tuberculosis, a list of staff at risk should be drawn by the line manager. This list should only include staff who have had direct contact. The list should be sent to the Occupational Health Department and Infection Control Doctor who will assess the circumstances of the exposure incident and review the health care workers on the contact list. The Occupational Health Department will consult the occupational health notes of the individual included on the contact list to identify Heaf/BCG status and take appropriate action.

VACCINATION AGAINST HEPATITIS B

All medical, dental, nursing and ancillary staff who have direct contact with patients' blood and secretions should be offered hepatitis B vaccine. The normal schedule is three doses of recombinant hepatitis B vaccine given at 0, 1 and 6 months. A test for serum antibodies to hepatitis B must be performed at 2-4 months after the end of the course. An antibody level of 100 miU/ml is considered to be protective. Poor antibody response (<10 miU /ml) may indicate that the person may have been exposed previously and could be a carrier of hepatitis B surface (HBsAg) or hepatitis e antigen (HBeAg). These individual should be counselled with regard to their work-related risk of infection and may be tested for markers of past infection or carriage of hepatitis B infection, at the discretion of the Consultant in the Occupational Health Medicine. An antibody response between 10 and 100 miU/ml indicates an unsatisfactory response to the vaccination and a fourth dose of the vaccine is required and antibody level checked at 2 month interval. An antibody level of more than 500miU/ml ia a good response to the vaccine and a booster is probably is not required for five years.

Staff accepting the offer of hepatitis B vaccine must sign an acceptance form indicating their agreement to complete the course. If for some reason the individual does not wish to receive the vaccine, he or she must sign a disclaimer section of the form. The Consultant in Occupational Health Medicine will re-evaluate the individual's risk of acquiring infection or transmission and the individual may not be allowed to carry out exposure prone procedures.

Any health care worker who performs exposure prone procedure and who has not been immunized should be tested for presence of hepatitis B surface(HBsAg) as soon as possible. This may mean testing before immunization has been completed. All staff who are HBsAg positive **must** cease exposure prone procedures until their HBeAg has been established. If the health care worker is HBeAg positive they must not be allowed to perform exposure procedures until they have been successfully treated with interferon alpha and their e antigen negative status is sustained for 12 months after cessation of treatment.

Blood samples taken from health care workers for the purpose of testing for current hepatitis B infection or response to vaccine should be taken directly by the Occupational Health Department.

MANAGEMENT OF SHARPS INJURY

The aim of this policy is to minimize the risk of infection in the health care setting from blood-borne pathogens which are most commonly involved in occupational transmission, ie hepatitis (B &C) and HIV infection. Guidance is also given on the procedures for dealing with sharps injury from contaminated sharps instruments and from other occupational exposure incidents which cause contamination of eye, mouth, skin cuts or abrasions from splashes, or spills of blood or high risk body fluids or tissues. The Department of Occupational Health Medicine has an overall responsibility for implementing, monitoring and co-ordinating the policy.

It is the responsibility of each head of department to ensure that their staff are aware of the content of the policy in order that each health care worker may initiate the appropriate post-exposure management. The procedure should be followed even if staff have been vaccinated against hepatitis B vaccine.

Whilst action may be taken to minimise the consequence of accidental exposure to blood-borne pathogens, it is in the interest of every health care worker to ensure that they employ safe techniques to prevent accidental exposure to

Table 6.1 – HBV prophylaxis for reported exposure incidents.

HBV status of person exposed	Significant exposure			Non-significant exposure	
	HBsAg positive source	**Unknown source**	**HBsAg negative source**	**Continued risk**	**No further risk**
≤1 dose HB vaccine pre-exposure	Accelerated course of HB vaccine* HBIG × 1	Accelerated course of HB vaccine*	Initiate course of HB vaccine	Initiate course of HB vaccine	No HBV prophylaxis Reassure
≥2 doses HB vaccine pre-exposure (anti-HBs not known)	One dose of HB vaccine followed by second dose one month later	One dose of HB vaccine	Finish course of HB vaccine	Finish course of HB vaccine	No HBV prophylaxis Reassure
Known responder to HB vaccine (anti-HBs ≥10miU/ml)	Booster dose of HB vaccine	Consider booster dose of HB vaccine	Consider booster dose of HB vaccine	Consider booster dose of HB vaccine	No HBV prophylaxis Reassure
Known non-responder to HB vaccine (anti-HBs <10miU/ml 2-4 months post-vaccination)	HBIG × 1 Consider booster dose of HB vaccine	HBIG × 1 Consider booster dose of HB vaccine	No HBIG Consider booster dose of HB vaccine	No HBIG Consider booster dose of HB vaccine	No HBV prophylaxis Reassure

* An accelerated course of vaccine consists of doses spaced at 0, 1 and 2 months. A booster dose is given at 12 months to those at continuing risk of exposure to HBV.

(Reproduced with permission from the *Communicable Disease Report* **2**(9): R97-101, 1992).

themselves and to others. Any health care worker who identifies a practice which they consider unsafe should inform their line manager so that remedial action may be taken to prevent injury or accident.

In cases of exposure to blood or body fluids the following procedures should be followed:

- Encourage the affected area of skin to bleed for few seconds.
- Do not suck the puncture site.
- Rinse immediately under running water and wash with soap and water and then with alcoholic/chlorhexidine solution ("Hibisol").
- Do not scrub. Rinse and dry.

If the spillage of blood and body fluid has occurred on intact skin then the effected area should be rinsed immediately under running water and washed with soap and water. Do not scrub. Rinse and dry. Exposed mucous membrane or conjunctive should be irrigated immediately with copious amounts of water using either running tap water or an eyewash bottle.

Immediate contact procedures: Inform your line manager or head of the department of the incident and ***immediately*** contact the Occupational Health Department or, out of hours, the Accident and Emergency department, according to the local policy. They will see the member of staff and advise on treatment. Ensure that the Accident Report Form is filled in. The Occupational Health or Accident and Emergency department will assess the member of staff and initiate investigation, treatment and counselling, where required.

In all cases of significant exposure, 10 ml clotted blood is taken (regardless of any previously documented serological test results) from the exposed individual and the serum stored (ideally at -70°C) for a minimum of 2 years. The individual should be assured that their blood will not be tested in any way without their consent. This is because it may be helpful to have access to stored serum should the person exposed subsequently be found to have serological evidence of blood-borne infection. Subsequent samples of blood from the health care worker should be obtained by the Consultant in Occupational Health Department depending of the incident history .

In cases where the patient can be identified, request the ward doctor to take a 10 ml clotted sample for immediate testing for hepatitis B surface antigen (HBsAg) from the source patient. If the HBsAg of the source is known at the time of incident, immediate HBsAg testing of the sample will not be necessary. It is not recommended, for the present, that post-exposure management of occupational exposure incidents should include routine testing against hepatitis C (anti-HCV) of a blood specimen from the identifiable patient source.

A risk assessment for the HIV infection must be made by the clinical team responsible for the patient's care. If suspected, the blood for HIV antibody testing must be taken only with the patient's ***informed consent*** (see page 137).

Decision about the need for the hepatitis prophylaxis is based on the immune status of the individual health care worker (Table 6.1 see page 153) and, if hepatitis B Immunoglobulin is considered necessary, it should be given as soon as possible, ie within 24 hours of the incident.

Occupational exposure and prophylaxis to HIV: If the nature of the exposure is thought to be HIV, the Consultant in the Occupational Health Department or microbiologist/virologist must be consulted urgently for advice and treatment. Accidental exposure to HIV infection in the health care setting should be reported to the Communicable Disease Surveillance Centre, London, in strict confidence, by the Consultant in Occupational Health Medicine.

An international case-control study of health care workers with percutaneous occupational exposure to HIV found that treatment after exposure with zidovudine reduced the probability of infection. The Centres for Disease Control recommend prophylaxis with three drugs (Zidovudine+Lamivudine+ Indinavir) for the highest risk exposures, with two drugs (Zidovudine+Lamivudine) for lower risk exposures, and no treatment for the lowest risk exposures (see reference). In the UK, the final recommendations for chemoprophylaxis with antiretroviral prophylaxis will be published in 1997 by the Department of Health Expert Advisory Group on AIDS.

Drug combinations should be guided by knowledge of the index patient's previous treatment. Prophylaxis should be given within one hour, after exposure; this requires health care facilities to have a system available to assist exposed health care workers which is available 24 hours a day. The risk of toxicity in each case must be balanced against the relatively low rate of infection after the average percutaneous exposure.

References and further reading

A Working Party of the PHLS Salmonella. The prevention of human transmission of gastrointestinal infections, infestations and bacterial intoxications. *Communicable Disease Report* 1995;**5**:R158-172.

Department of Health Welsh Office. *The Prevention and Control of Tuberculosis in the United Kingdom: Recommendations for the prevention and control of tuberculosis at local level* London: Department of Health, 1996.

Joint Tuberculosis Committee of the British Thoracic Society. Control and prevention of tuberculosis in the United Kingdom: Code of Practice 1994. *Thorax* 1994; **49**:1193-1200.

UK Department of Health. *AIDS/HIV-infected health care worker: guidance on the management of the infected health care workers*. London: Department of Health, 1994.

PHLS Hepatitis subcommittee. Exposure to hepatitis B virus: guidance on post-exposure prophylaxis. *Communicable Disease Report* 1992;**2**:R97-101.

UK Department of Health. *Protecting health care workers and patients from hepatitis B*. London: Department of Health, 1994.

NHS Executive. Addendum to HSG(93)40. *Protecting health care workers and patients from hepatitis B*. EL (96)77. September 1996.

British Medical Association. *A code of practice for implementation of the UK hepatitis B immunisation guidelines for the protection of patients and staff*. London: British Medical Association, 1995.

Hepatitis C virus: guidance on the risks and current management of occupational exposure. *Communicable Disease Report* 1993; **3**: R135-139.

BMA Board of Science and Education. *A guide to hepatitis C*. London: British Medical Association, 1996.

Gerberding JL. Management of occupational exposures to blood-borne viruses. *New England Journal of Medicine* 1995; **332**:444-451.

Rhodes RS, Bell DM. Prevention of transmission of blood-borne pathogens. *The Surgical Clinics of North America* 1995; **75(6)**: 1047-1241.

Centres for Disease Control. Case-control Study of HIV seroconversin in health care workers after percutaneous exposure to HIV infected blood -France, United Kingdom and United States, January 1988 - August 1994. *Morbidity and Mortality Weekly Report* 1995; **44**: 929-933.

Update: Provision Public Health Service Recommendations for Chemoprophylaxis after Occupational Exposure to HIV. *Morbidity and Mortality Weekly Report* 1995; **45**: 468- 472.

Department of Health Welsh, Scottish Office Department of Health, DHSS (N. Ireland) *Immunisation against Infectious Disease*. London: HMSO, 1996.

Cardo DM, Bell DM. Bloodborne Pathogen Transmission in Health Care Workers: Risks and Prevention Strategies. *Infectious Disease Clinics of North America* 1997; **11**: 331-346.

Doebbeling BN, Protecting the Healthcare Worker from Infection and Injury. In: Wenzel RP, ed. *Prevention and Control of Nosocomial Infections*. 3rd ed. Baltimore: Williams & Wilkins 1997: 397-435.

7

HAND WASHING AND HAND DISINFECTION

The spread of infection by direct contact from health care workers' hands is the most common means by which infection is transmitted between personnel and patients within the health care setting. Hand washing is therefore considered to be one of the most important procedures in the prevention of cross-infection in health care facilities. The efficacy of a hand wash depends on the technique and the time taken.

Organisms present on the hands may be divided into two categories:

Resident organisms

These microorganisms are normal flora of the skin and include coagulase-negative staphylococci (mainly *Staph. epidermidis*), members of the genus *Corynebacterium* (commonly called diphtheroids) and *Propionibacterium* spp. They are usually deep seated in the epidermis and are not easily removed by a single hand washing procedure. They rarely cause infection apart from during implant surgery and at intravenous sites.

Transient organisms

These microorganisms are those that are not part of the normal flora and represent recent contaminations which usually survive only for a limited period of time. They are acquired during contact with the infected/colonized patient or the environment and are easily removed by a good hand washing technique. The transient flora includes most of the organisms responsible for cross-infection, eg Gram-negative bacilli (*E. coli, Klebsiella* and *Pseudomonas* spp.), *Salmonella* spp., *Staph.aureus* and viruses, eg rotaviruses.

ROUTINE HAND WASHING

Routine hand washing will render the hands socially clean and remove transient microorganisms provided that an effective technique is used.

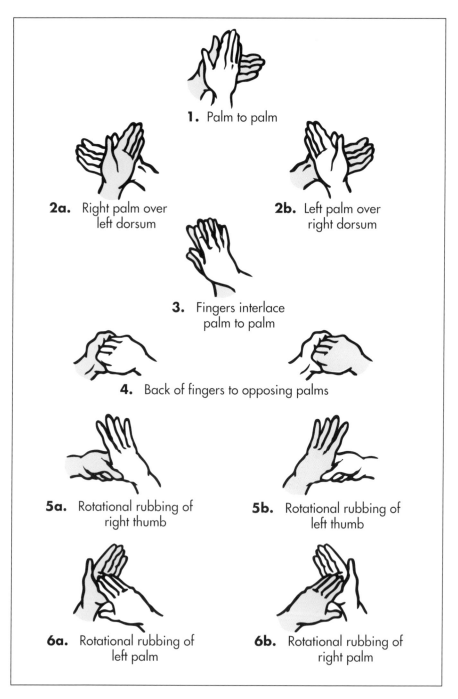

1. Palm to palm

2a. Right palm over left dorsum

2b. Left palm over right dorsum

3. Fingers interlace palm to palm

4. Back of fingers to opposing palms

5a. Rotational rubbing of right thumb

5b. Rotational rubbing of left thumb

6a. Rotational rubbing of left palm

6b. Rotational rubbing of right palm

Figure 7.1 – Figures showing steps in hand washing technique.
(From Ayliffe GAJ. *et al.* 1978.)

Procedure

1. Wet hands and forearms.

2. Apply sufficient plain, non-microbial (bar or liquid) soap to the hands to obtain a good lather.

3. Rub vigorously to form a lather on the surface of the hands for at least 10-15 seconds.

4. The hands should then be thoroughly rinsed under running water for a further 10-15 seconds.

5. Dry thoroughly using good quality paper towels.

Hands should be washed :

- before and after a work shift.
- before and after each nursing contact.
- after contact with blood, body fluids, secretion and excretion.
- after handling soiled or contaminated equipment or linen.
- before eating, drinking or handling food, including serving meals or drinks or administering drugs.
- after using the toilet.

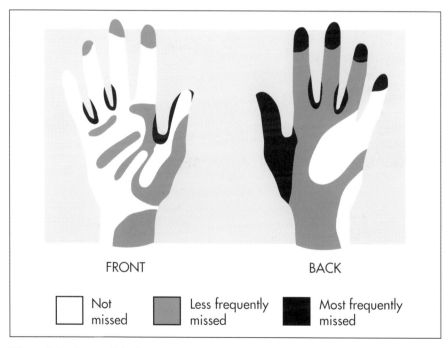

FRONT   BACK

☐ Not missed   ▨ Less frequently missed   ■ Most frequently missed

Figure 7.2 – Parts of the hands most frequently missed during hand washing
(Reproduced with permission from Taylor LJ. An evaluation of handwashing techniques. *Nursing Times* 1978; **74**: 54-55).

HYGIENIC HAND DISINFECTION

Hygienic hand disinfection will remove and kill most transient microorganisms. An antiseptic hand wash preparation is used.

Procedure

1. Wet hands and forearms.

2. Apply 3-5 ml of antiseptic solution into cupped hands.

3. Rub vigorously to form a lather on all surfaces of the hands and forearms for at least one minute.

4. The hands should then be thoroughly rinsed under running water for 10-15 seconds, applying friction over all hand surfaces.

5. Rinse and then dry thoroughly.

It should be used :

- during outbreaks of infection where contact with blood and body fluids or in situations where microbial contamination is likely to occur.
- in high risk areas, eg patients in isolation, Intensive Care and Special Care Baby Unit.
- before performing an invasive procedure.
- before and after touching wounds, urethral or IV catheters.
- before wearing and after removing gloves.

HYGIENIC HAND RUB

An alternative method of hand disinfection is the application of 3-5 ml of a fast-acting antiseptic (eg, alcoholic hand rub ("Hibisol") containing glycerol as an emollient to prevent excessive drying of hands) into cupped hands and by using the defined technique, the hands are rubbed until they are dried. Alcoholic hand rubs do not cleanse and therefore it is important that hands should be cleaned with soap and water first in the presence of visible contamination. This method is convenient since dispensers for hand rubs can easily be made available wherever necessary. It is also a rapid and effective alternative to hand washing in areas where a wash hand basin is not readily available, eg in the community or when return to a wash hand basin is impractical, for example during a ward round where there is a need for rapid hand disinfection.

SURGICAL HAND DISINFECTION

Surgical hand washing (surgical scrub) requires the removal and killing of transient microorganisms and substantial reduction and suppuration of the resident flora of the surgical team for the duration of operation in case a surgical glove is punctured or torn. Ensure that fingernails are kept short and clean all the time. Wrist watches and jewellery should be removed before surgical hand disinfection.

Procedure

1. Turn the taps on using the elbows and adjust the flow of water and temperature of the water.

2. Wet hands and forearms.

3. Apply an antiseptic, eg chlorhexidine or povidone iodine, detergent preparation from an elbow operated pump dispenser.

4. Lather hands, wrists and forearms for one minute, keeping them above elbow level and rinse thoroughly under running water. Clean finger nails and remove ingrained dirt with a manicure stick held under running water or use a sterile nail brush to clean nails and subungual spaces (but not the skin to prevent skin damage) only at the beginning of the operation list.

5. The hand washing procedure is then repeated for two more minutes. The hands, wrists and forearms are then rinsed thoroughly under running water, making sure that fingertips should always point upward, with elbows down, to avoid recontamination of clean fingers and hands by water running down from contaminated proximal areas.

6. The technique of drying is very important. A separate, sterile towel is used for each arm, moving from fingertips to elbow using a dabbing action.

7. The towel is discarded and the procedure is repeated for the other arm.

8. When both hands, wrists and forearms are thoroughly dry, the individual is ready to gown and glove.

Some surgeons may prefer to disinfect their hands using antiseptic detergent, as described in the surgical hand washing technique, at the beginning of an operating list and then continue with an application of alcoholic solution for subsequent operations. If alcoholic preparation is used, two applications of 5 ml each is applied to cover the entire surface of hands and forearms and rubbed to dryness. Chlorhexidine has a good residual effect, but the alcoholic solutions have a greater immediate and prolonged effect even without an added antiseptic.

GENERAL COMMENTS

Soap: For general patient care a plain, non-microbial bar of soap should be used. Small bars are recommended so they can be changed frequently. The soap should be kept dry (in a soap rack or on a magnet or ring) to promote drainage of water to avoid contamination with the microorganisms which grow in moist conditions. Liquid soap products should be stored in closed containers and dispensed from disposable containers. The dispensers should be regularly cleaned and maintained.

Antiseptics: A range of products are available, but chlorhexidine, povidone iodine, alcohols and triclosan are commonly used. Examples include 4% Chlorhexidine gluconate-detergent ("Hibiscrub"), Povidone iodine solution containing 0.75% available iodine ("Betadine"), 0.5% Chlorhexidine gluconate with 70% isopropyl alcohol ("Hibisol") or 2% Triclosan in a tenside base ("Aquasept").

Nail Brush: A soft nail brush should not be used routinely other than possibly for cleaning the nails and subungual spaces prior to the first operation of the day. Frequent and vigorous use of a nail brush may damage the skin, encouraging the proliferation and persistence of microorganisms on the skin. Nail brushes used should either be sterile single-use disposable or sterilized by the hospital CSSD. Never soak nail brushes in disinfectant solution.

Gloves: A glove is not always an impermeable barrier but they may reduce the transfer of microorganisms. They should not be regarded as a substitute for hand washing.

If gloves are worn in an outbreak situation, it is important that the same gloves must not be worn from one patient to another, or between clean and dirty procedures on the same patient. Hands must be washed after removing gloves; wearing gloves does not obviate the need for hand washing. Nails should be kept short to allow thorough cleaning of the hands and to prevent tears in gloves.

Lotions: Lotions may be used to prevent skin drying associated with hand washing. They should be supplied in small, individual use containers that are not refilled.

Some types of hand creams and lotions may interact with antiseptics used for hand washing and on the integrity of gloves. Some are also responsible for skin sensitization. Therefore, only suitable hand cream or lotion should be used.

PRACTICAL POINTS

- Unless the water is turned off by an automatic device, the water should be turned off using a paper towel rather than bare fingers or hands in order to avoid recontamination of hands after hand washing.

- In wash basins no plug is necessary, since hands should be washed only under running water.

- Similar concentrations of the antiseptic agent in different products does not necessarily imply equal effectiveness, therefore new products should be tested before introduction.

- Any preparations used for hand washing or disinfection must be acceptable to the user and should not damage the skin on repeated use. If the preparation is not accepted by staff it will not be used. Therefore, it is recommended that a trial is done in some areas to assess the acceptability by staff.

- Any type of cloth towels are *not* recommended for use in health care facilities. Only good quality paper towels within easy reach of a sink but beyond splash contamination should be used.

References and further reading

Larson EL. APIC guideline for handwashing and hand antisepsis in health care settings. *American Journal of Infection Control* 1995; **23:** 251-269.

Taylor LJ. An evaluation of handwashing techniques. *Nursing Times* 1978; **74:** 54-55 (part I), 108-110 (part II).

Rotter ML. Hand Washing and Hand Disinfection. In: Mayhall CG, ed. *Hospital Epidemiology and Infection Control. Baltimore:* Williams & Wilkins, 1996: 1052-1068.

Reybrouck G. Hand washing and hand disinfection. *Journal of Hospital Infection* 1986; **8:** 5-23.

Larson E. Guidelines for use of topical antimicrobial agents. *American Journal of Infection Control* 1988; **16(6):** 253-266.

Ayliffe GAJ, Babb JR, Davies JG, Lilly HA. Hand disinfection: a comparison of various agents in laboratory and ward studies. *Journal of Hospital Infection* 1988; **11:** 226-246.

Rotter ML. Hand Washing, Hand Disifection, and Skin Disinfection. In: Wenzel RP, ed. *Prevention and Control of Nosocomial Infections*. 3rd ed. Baltimore: Williams & WIlkins 1997; 691-709.

8

PREVENTION OF INFECTION ASSOCIATED WITH INTRAVENOUS THERAPY

Insertion of an intravenous catheter either peripheral or central is one of the most commonly performed medical procedures for various medical indications. Among various other complications, catheter-related sepsis is one of the most important. The risk of infection associated with intravenous (IV) catheters varies depending on the type of device used. For example, the incidence of catheter-related bloodstream infection associated with short-term Teflon IV catheters is much less than long-term central venous catheters.

An intravenous catheter is a foreign body which produces a reaction in the host consisting of a film of fibrinous material (biofilm) on the inner and outer surfaces of the catheter. This biofilm may become colonized by microorganisms and will be protected from host defence mechanisms. Infection usually follows colonization of the biofilm causing local sepsis, septic thrombophlebitis or, in some cases systemic infection, eg bacteraemia or septicaemia.

Sources of infection may be:

Intrinsic

This is due to contamination or faulty sterilization of fluids during manufacture. It is usually due to Gram-negative organisms growing in the infusate, such as *Klebsiella, Enterobacter* or *Pseudomonas* spp.

Extrinsic

This is due to contamination of the IV catheter during the insertion, administration of the fluid or from the hands of the operator. However, the most important reservoirs of pathogens causing catheter-related infection are the insertion site and the hub. It is mainly due to microorganisms residing on the patient's skin, eg *Staph. epidermidis, Staph.aureus* and diphtheroids.

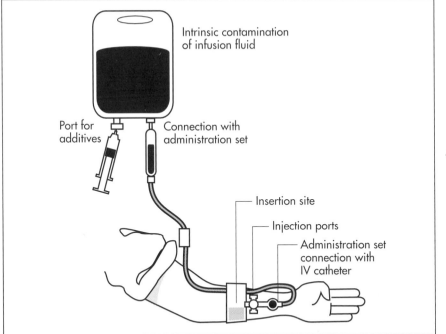

Figure 8.1 – Points of access for microbial contamination in infusion therapy.

INSERTION OF PERIPHERAL INTRAVENOUS CATHETER

Ensure that the patient is in a comfortable position and aware of the nature of the procedure as this will reduce anxiety.

Procedure

1. Collect all necessary equipment.

2. Operator should wash hands thoroughly with soap and running water for 15-20 seconds and dry hands thoroughly on a paper towel. An antiseptic-detergent or alcohol hand rub is preferred, if available, and should be used before insertion of a catheter requiring a cut down.

3. Select an appropriate site, avoiding bony prominences and joints.

4. Disinfect the IV insertion site with a 70% isopropyl alcohol impregnated swab for at least 30 seconds prior to venepuncture and allow the insertion site to dry before inserting the catheter.

   The venepuncture site should not be touched once the vein has been selected and the skin prepared; avoid touching the shaft of the catheter with fingers during insertion.

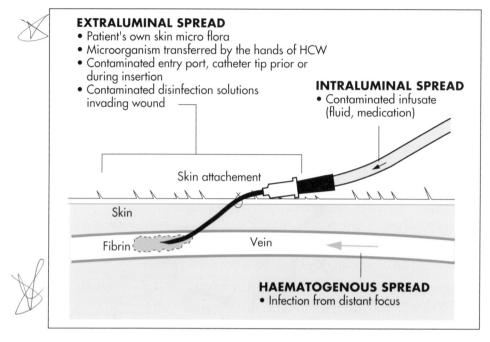

EXTRALUMINAL SPREAD
- Patient's own skin micro flora
- Microorganism transferred by the hands of HCW
- Contaminated entry port, catheter tip prior or during insertion
- Contaminated disinfection solutions invading wound

INTRALUMINAL SPREAD
- Contaminated infusate (fluid, medication)

Skin attachement

Skin

Fibrin

Vein

HAEMATOGENOUS SPREAD
- Infection from distant focus

Figure 8.2 – Sources of microbial contamination in patients with intravenous catheter.
(Reproduced with modification from Bennett JV, Brachman PS. *Hospital Infection* 3 rd. *ed*. Boston, Little Brown, 1992)

5. Select a catheter that will fit easily into the vein. The correct sized catheter reduces trauma and congestion of the vein.

6. Insert the catheter as swiftly and as aseptically as possible using "no touch" technique. Do not attempt repeated insertions with the same catheter. If the first insertion is not successful the procedure should be repeated with a new catheter.

7. Look out for flashback of blood and then advance the catheter slowly.

8. Secure the catheter with an appropriate sterile gauze or transparent adhesive dressing to prevent movement of catheter. Label the site with the insertion date.

9. Connect up the intravenous administration set.

10. Clean around the site with a 70% isopropyl alcohol impregnated swab.

11. Ensure that all sharps are safely discarded into a sharps bin.

12. Wash and dry hands.

INSERTION OF CENTRAL VENOUS CATHETER

The insertion of a central venous catheter is an aseptic procedure. Face masks and caps are not necessary. Long sleeved gowns or aprons should be worn. The hands must be washed with an antiseptic detergent hand wash preparation for one minute and sterile gloves should be worn.

Procedure

1. Collect all necessary equipment.

2. The operator should wash hands using an antiseptic-detergent or an alcohol hand rub.

3. Disinfect site with antiseptic alcoholic chlorhexidine, or alcoholic povidone iodine solution, with friction for at least 3 minutes prior to venepuncture. Allow site to dry before inserting catheter.

4. Surround the site with large sheet of sterile drapes.

5. Insert the central venous catheter as swiftly as possible maintaining "no touch" technique throughout the procedure.

6. Blood should be aspirated freely to ensure that the catheter is in a vascular space before injecting fluid. Position of CVP line must be checked by the x-ray.

7. Leave the site clean and dry after insertion.

8. Secure the catheter with an appropriate sterile dressing or clear semi-permeable dressing. Label the site with insertion date; insertion date should preferably be recorded in the patient's medical notes.

9. Connect up the intravenous administration set.

10. Ensure that all sharps are safely discarded into a sharps bin.

11. Wash and dry hands.

PRACTICAL POINTS

- IV catheter teams, consisting of highly trained staff to ensure stringent adherence to aseptic techniques during catheter insertion and later catheter manipulation, significantly reduce the risk of infection and are cost-effective.

- Remove any intravascular device as soon as its use is no longer clinically indicated, as the risk of infection increases with the length of time of catheterization. Therefore, all patients with intravenous catheters should be evaluated on a daily basis for evidence of catheter-related complications, ie tenderness, thrombosis, swelling, or signs of inflammation or infection. The insertion site should be palpated daily for tenderness through intact dressing.

- Antibiotic prophylaxis before or during catheter insertion is not recommended to prevent catheter colonization or bloodstream infection. Routine use of topical antimicrobial ointments are also not recommended at the site of catheter insertion.

- The catheter should not be inserted into an area of inflammation or infection and must be removed and re-sited, if required.

- Any catheter inserted without proper asepsis, ie those inserted in an emergency, should be removed and re-sited at the earliest opportunity, ie within 24 hours.

- Replace IV tubing, including piggyback tubing and stopcocks, no more frequently than at 72 hour intervals, unless clinically indicated.

- In adults, use an upper extremity site in preference to one on a lower extremity for catheter insertion. Transfer a catheter inserted in a low extremity site to an upper extremity site as soon as the latter is available. In paediatric patients, insert catheters into a scalp, hand or foot site in preference to a leg, arm or antecubital fossa site.

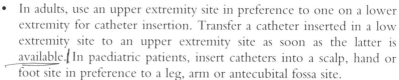

- In adults, replace short, peripheral venous catheters, and rotate peripheral venous sites every 48-72 hours to minimise the risk of phlebitis.

- Use a single-lumen central venous catheter, unless multiple ports are essential for the management of the patient.

- Use subclavian rather than jugular or femoral sites for central venous catheter placement unless medically contraindicated.

- Replace tubing used to administer blood, blood products, or lipid emulsions within 24 hours of initiating the infusion.

- Wipe the outer hub of the catheter with a 70% isopropyl alcohol impregnated swab before attaching the administration set. The luer lock should be kept clean and dry as possible.

- If there is a strong suspicion of infection, the line should be removed and the distal 3-5 cm should be sent to the bacteriology laboratory for culture in a sterile container. Blood culture, ideally from peripheral veins, and a wound swab should be taken from the site of insertion. If microbiological investigation proves catheter infection then the catheter should be removed and an alternative site chosen for re-insertion. It should be emphasized that intravenous devices cannot be "sterilized" with antibiotics and should be removed if the patient develops infection. In cases of proven catheter-related sepsis, appropriate antibiotics should be given before fresh catheter insertion to prevent recolonization of new IV lines. The choice of antibiotic will depend on the sensitivity of the microorganism; for blind therapy the medical microbiologist should be contacted for advice.

References and further reading

Hospital Infection Control Practices Advisory Committee. Part I. Intravascular device-related infections: an overview. Part II. Recommendation for the prevention of nosocomial intravascular device-related infections. *American Journal of Infection Control* 1996; **24:** 262-293.

Mermel LA. Infection related to intravascular devices. In: Olmsted RN, (ed). *APIC Infection Control and Applied Epidemiology: Principles and Practice.* St Louis: Mosby, 1996: 9.1-9.6.

Elliott TSJ, Faroqui MH, Armstrong, RF, Hanson GC. Guidelines for good practice in central venous catheterization. *The Journal of Hospital Infection* 1994; **28**(3): 163-176.

Widmer AF. Intravenous-Related Infections. In: Wenzel RP. ed. *Prevention and Control of Nosocomial Infections.* 3rd ed. Batimore: Williams & Wilkins 1997; 771-805

Maki DG. Infections due to infusion therapy. In: Bennet JV, Brachman PS, (eds). *Hospital Infections.* 3rd ed. Boston: Little Brown, 1993: 849-898.

9

PREVENTION OF INFECTION ASSOCIATED WITH URINARY CATHETER

About 10% of hospitalized patients have an indwelling catheter, of which 20-25% develop Urinary Tract Infection (UTI). It is estimated that hospital acquired UTIs account for 40% of hospital-acquired infections. Most of these are associated with instrumentation, particularly indwelling catheterization. Most patients will have asymptomatic bacteriuria or mild symptoms like suprapubic pain and urethral burning that tend to be self-limiting when the catheter is removed. However, some patients will develop severe infections, pyelonephritis or septicaemia. Therefore, it is important that indwelling catheters should only be used when there is a clear medical indication. They should preferably not be used solely for the management of urinary incontinence. Alternatives to indwelling catheters are intermittent catheterization with associated infection risk of UTI ranging from 0.5-8%.

The incidence of infection is directly related to the duration of catheterization; 50% of patients are infected by day 15 of catheterization, and almost 100% by 1 month. Therefore, catheterization should be avoided, if possible, and if indicated it should be removed as soon as possible, preferably within 5 days.

Catheter size relates to the circumference of the catheter. The smallest size consistent for confident insertion and satisfactory drainage should be used as the narrower size or gauge catheters are less likely to irritate the urethra to predispose to infection.

PROCEDURE

With the inherent risk of introducing infection to the urinary tract, catheterization must be performed as an aseptic procedure and the aseptic technique should be maintained throughout the procedure. Explaining the nature of the procedure to the patient will reduce anxiety.

1. All equipment used must be sterile. Lay out the top of the trolley making sure all items required are open and accessible.

2. Hands must be washed thoroughly with an antiseptic hand wash preparation.

3. Sterile gloves must be worn and a "no-touch" aseptic technique should be used.

4. The peri-urethral area should be thoroughly cleaned, preferably with an antiseptic, eg chlorhexidine solution to minimize introduction of skin and faecal flora into the bladder. In a male, grasp the distal shaft of the penis and retract the foreskin. Cleanse the glans with a disinfectant/detergent preparation. In a female, separate the labia and cleanse the vulva using front to back technique.

5. Sterile anaesthetic (1-2% lignocaine/chlorhexidine) gel can be instilled into the urethra to minimise pain. If used, allow 5 minutes for it to take anaesthetic effect before catheterization.

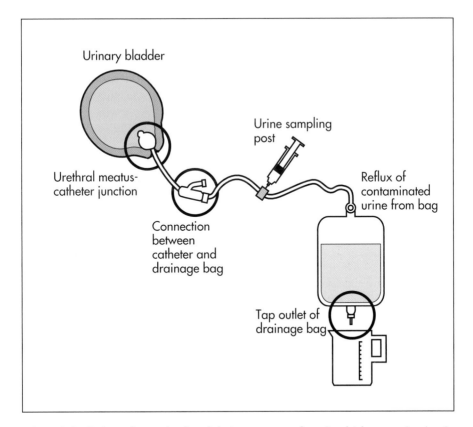

Figure 9.1 – Points of entry in closed drainage system for microbial contamination in catheterized patient.

6. Gently insert the catheter and advance it by holding the inner sterile sleeve avoiding contact with non–sterile surfaces. Ideally, the "no touch" technique should be used in which the operator has no contact with the sterile shaft of the catheter.

7. Inflate the balloon by instilling the manufacturer's recommended amount of sterile water.

8. Attach a sterile urine drainage bag.

9. Connect the catheter to the closed drainage bag and hang it below the level of the bed to stop reflux. The bag must be supported in the drainage stand to allow free flow of urine and prevent the bag touching the floor.

10. Secure the catheter to the patient's thigh to prevent movement and urethral meatal ulceration.

GENERAL COMMENTS

Drainage bag: Only a sterile bag which facilitates a closed system of drainage should be used which should be fixed on a portable stand. The bag and tubing should at all times be below the level of the bladder so that the flow can be continuously maintained by gravity. The spout from the tap should be completely emptied to minimise a build-up of organisms in the stagnant urine. Routine use of antiseptics and hydrogen peroxide in the drainage bag are not recommended.

Emptying the drainage bag: Extreme care must be taken when emptying the drainage bag to prevent cross-infection. The hands are washed and non–sterile disposable gloves must be worn before emptying each bag. The bag should be emptied via the drainage tap at the bottom of the bag. When the bag is empty, the tap should be closed securely and wiped with a tissue. If the bag does not have a tap, replace it when full using an aseptic technique. Do not reconnect a used bag. Wash and dry hands thoroughly after touching the drainage bag.

A separate urine collecting receptacle must be used for each patient and each bag should be emptied separately as required. For purposes of measuring urinary output, an integral measuring device is necessary. The urine receptacle should be heat disinfected and stored dry after each use. Single-use disposable receptacles may be used. After emptying the receptacle, the gloves should be discarded and hands washed and dried thoroughly.

Specimen collection: Do not disconnect the drainage bag to obtain a sample as this causes interruption to the closed drainage system and may pose a risk of infection to the patient. If a sample of urine is required for bacteriological examination, it should be obtained from a sampling port or sleeve. This must first be disinfected by wiping with a 70% isopropyl alcohol impregnated swab. The sample may then be aspirated using a sterile needle and syringe and transferred into a sterile container. ***Do not*** obtain a sample for bacteriological culture from the drainage bag.

Bladder irrigation: Routine irrigation of bladder (bladder washout) with chlorhexidine or other antiseptics are not effective in prevention of infection and should not be performed. They rarely eradicate organisms, may introduce infection, can cause inflammation of the bladder wall and, therefore, increase the likelihood of systemic invasion. They may also cause damage to the catheter.

If the catheter becomes obstructed and can be kept open only by frequent irrigation the catheter should be changed as it is likely that the catheter itself is contributing to obstruction.

Prophylaxis and treatment with antibiotics: Routine use of prophylactic antibiotic administration in catheterized patients is ***not*** recommended because of its tendency to encourage the emergence of resistant organisms. Long term antibiotic prophylaxis is ineffective and predisposes to infection with resistant organisms. Treatment of asymptomatic bacteriuria (ie, significant bacteriuria in absence of clinical symptoms) in patients who require continued catheterization is also not indicated. Treat patients with antibiotics only if there is evidence of clinical infection. Treatment of catheter associated urinary tract infections in patients with long-term catheters may be difficult without removal or changing of the catheter because of the build up of organisms in a biofilm on the internal catheter surface. The use of antibiotic in the presence of the catheter often results in superinfection with a more resistant strain of bacteria. After the catheter is removed, in most patients the bacteriuria spontaneously resolves; if treatment is indicated it is only for those cases in which the bacteriuria has persisted after catheter removal and in which there are no underlying anatomic or physiologic barriers to eradication of the bacteriuria.

Patients with infected urine at the time of catheterization or operation should be treated with appropriate antibiotics according to the antibiotic sensitivity of the organism. If antibiotic sensitivity testing is not available, blind antibiotic treatment can be given according to the local antibiotic policy, or advice sought from a medical microbiologist.

PRACTICAL POINTS

- If the catheter will not pass any part of the urethra with gentle pressure, or if a trace of blood is seen on the catheter tip on withdrawal, do not persevere or push harder, as serious damage may ensue. In this case, seek help from a more experienced colleague.

- The most effective measure to prevent clinically significant infection, catheter blockage and bleeding is to ensure optimal fluid intake and urinary output.

- Catheterized patients with multi-resistant microorganisms should be nursed in a side room with en suite toilet facilities and implement infection control precautions as advised by a member of the Infection Control Team.

References and further reading

Falkiner FR. The insertion and management of indwelling urethral catheter-minimizing the risk of infection. *Journal of Hospital Infection* 1993; **25:** 79-90.

Stickler DJ, Zimakoff. Complications of urinary tract infections associated with devices used for long-term bladder management. *Journal of Hospital Infection* 1994; **28:** 177-194.

Warren JW. Urinary Infections. Wenzel RP, ed. *Prevention and Control of Nosocomial Infections.* 3rd ed. Baltimore: Williams & Wilkins 1997; 822-840.

Stamm WE. Catheter-associated urinary tract infection: epidemiology, pathogenesis and prevention. *American Journal of Medicine* 1991; **91**(Supplement 3B): 655-715.

10

PREVENTION OF NOSOCOMIAL PNEUMONIA

Nosocomial pneumonia is the second most common type of hospital-acquired infection and is associated with a mortality rate between 20-50%. Compared to non–ventilated patients, the risk of pneumonia is increased at least 7 to 10 fold in patients following surgery or in intensive care who require mechanical ventilation. This is due to mechanical and chemical injury to the ciliated epithelial membrane of the respiratory tract which promotes colonization and aspiration of bacteria from the oropharynx or stomach into the tracheo-bronchial tree. Other risk factors are outlined in Table 10.1.

Approximately 30% of patients who are hospitalized, but are not critically ill or intubated, become colonized within 48 hours of admission, often with hospital-associated bacteria which are usually resistant to multiple antibiotics. The rate of colonization rises to 75% in the critically ill patients. Most cases of nosocomial pneumonia are caused by aerobic Gram-negative bacilli, ie *Pseudomonas aeruginosa, Klebsiella pneumonia, E. coli, Serratia marcescens, Citrobacter, Enterobacter* and *Acinetobacter* species. Gram-positive cocci *Staph. aureus. Strep. pneumonia* and *H. influenzae* can also cause post-operative pneumonia, particularly in patients with pre-existing pulmonary disease. Legionella may be acquired from hospital air conditioning systems or from water supplies, particularly in immunocompromised patients. Other organisms, eg respiratory syncytial and other viruses and fungi, eg *Candida albicans* and *Aspergillus fumigates* (associated with building work) may also cause nosocomial pneumonia.

Pneumocystis carinii causes pneumonia in immunosuppressed patients, particularly in AIDS patients. *Mycobacterium tuberculosis* and other atypical mycobacteria are also responsible for causing pneumonia.

The following measures should be adopted to prevent cross-infection and nosocomial pneumonia in hospitalized patients:

- Surveillance in the Intensive Care Unit. Introduce awareness programme in infection control to reduce nosocomial infection.

- Wash hands before and after procedures and patient contact.

- Wear gloves for contact with the respiratory secretions, devices, or environmental surfaces. Wash hands after removing gloves.

- If stress bleeding prophylaxis is considered necessary, consider an agent that does not raise the gastric pH. Sucralfate appears to be as effective as antacids and H_2 blockers but acts by a cytoprotective mechanism that does not block or significantly neutralise gastric acid secretion and is associated with a reduced infection rate.

- Pre-operatively encourage patient to stop smoking and resolve existing infection. Teach patient post-operative coughing exercise and breathing techniques.

Table 10.1 – Risk factors for oropharyngeal colonization and nosocomial pneumonia.

Extreme age (elderly or neonate)
Chronic disease or impaired immunity
Chronic lung disease
Existing cardiopulmonary disease
Immunosuppressive or cytotoxic drugs
Mechanical ventilation
Major injuries
Upper abdominal and thoracic surgery
Severe illness, eg septic shock
Aspiration
Tracheostomy, tracheal intubation
Achlorhydria, H_2 antagonist or antacids therapy
General anaesthesia
Depressed consciousness, eg coma, cerebrovascular accidents
Sedative or hypnotic drugs
Neuromuscular disease
Heavy smokers
Nasogastric tube
Prolonged hospitalization
Obesity or malnutrition
Prior infection or antimicrobial therapy

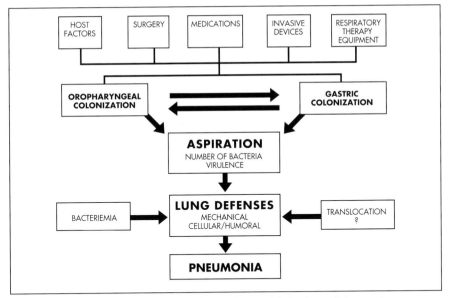

Figure 10.1 – Factors influencing colonization and infection of the respiratory tract. (Reproduced with permission from Craven *et al.* Nosocomial pneumonia in the 90's: update of the epidemiology and risk factors. *Semin Respir Infect* 1990; **5:** 157-192).

- Post-operatively turn patient to encourage postural drainage, encourage him/her to take deep breaths and cough. Mobilise early after operation. Judiciously control pain with analgesics and provide wound support.

- Nasogastric tube for enteral feeding may erode mucosal surface or block sinus ducts and is responsible for causing regurgitating gastric contents leading to aspiration. Assess nutritional status and remove nasogastric tube as clinically indicated.

- Maintain patient in an upright position (elevate patient's head to 30 - 45 degree angle) to reduce reflux and aspiration of gastric bacteria.

- ***Do not*** routinely administer antimicrobials for prophylaxis of pneumonia. Restrict widespread use of broad spectrum antibiotics.

- Educate staff in patient care and cleaning and disinfection of respiratory equipment.

- Perform tracheostomy under aseptic conditions.

- Selective decontamination of the oropharynx and gastrointestinal tract with use of oral or parenteral antibiotics in a critically ill or mechanically ventilated patient in the Intensive Care Unit is controversial.

Table 10.2 – Methods of prevention of nosocomial pneumonia.

Procedure / device	Intervention to decrease risk
Suction catheter	Single-use non-sterile disposal gloves should be worn for suctioning. Change suction catheter between patients and after each use.
Suction bottle	Use single-use disposable or if re-usable wash with detergent, dry and disinfect them using autoclave or disinfect them in washing machine.
Breathing circuit	Change mechanical ventilators circuit every 48 hours. Periodically drain breathing-tube condensation traps, taking care not to spill it down the patient's trachea; wash hands after the procedure.
Nebulizers	Change and reprocess device between patients by using sterilization or a high level of disinfection or use single-use disposable item. Fill with sterile water only.
Humidifiers	Clean and sterilize device between patients and fill with sterile water which must be changed every 24 hours or sooner, if necessary. Single-use disposable humidifiers are available but they are expensive.
Anaesthesia machine	After every patient, clean and then sterilize or subject to high-level liquid chemical disinfection or pasteurize re-usable components of breathing system or patient circuit according to the manufacturer's instructions for reprocessing.
Spirometry	Mouthpiece for each patient should be single-use disposable. Additional cleaning is indicated according manufacturer's recommendation.

References and further reading

Tablan OC, Anderson LF, Arden NH *et al*. Guideline for prevention of nosocomial pneumonia. *Infection Control and Hospital Epidemiology* 1994; **15:** 587-627.

George DL. Nosocomial pneumonia. In: Mayhall CG, (ed). *Hospital Epidemiology and Infection Control. Baltimore:* Williams & Wilkins, 1993:175-195.

Craven DE, Barber TW, Steger KA, Montecalvo MA. Nosocomial pneumonia in the 90's: update on epidemiology and risk factors. *Seminars in Respiratory Infection* 1990; **5:** 152-172.

Webb CW. Selective bowel decontamination in intensive care - a critical appraisal. *Reviews in Medical Microbiology* 1992; **3:** 202-210.

Mayhall CG. Nosocomial Pneumonia: Diagnisis and Prevention. *Infectious Disease Clinics of North America* 1997; **11(2):** 427-457.

Wiblin RT. Nosocomial Pneumonia In: Wenzel RP, (ed). *Prevention and Control of Nosocomial Infections*. 3rd ed. Baltimore: Williams & Wilkins 1997: 807-819.

11

PREVENTION OF SURGICAL WOUND INFECTION

Despite advances in the operative techniques and better understanding of the pathogenesis of wound infection, post-operative wound infection continues to be a major source of morbidity and mortality for patients undergoing operative procedures. It can account for up to 30% of hospital-acquired infection. The sources of infection may be endogenous (organisms acquired from patient's own body) or exogenous (organisms acquired from the environment). In order to minimise post-operative surgical wound infection, it is important to create a safe environment by controlling four main sources of infection, ie personnel, equipment, the environment and patient's risk factors.

The local manifestations of wound infection include one or more of the following: pain, erythema, induration, poor healing, dehiscence and presence of purulent drainage. Systematic manifestations commonly include fever and other signs of sepsis or bacteraemia.

PRE-OPERATIVE PATIENT CARE

Patients risk factors

Includes extreme age, obesity, malnutrition, certain concurrent disease or conditions, ie diabetes, malignancy, chronic chest or heart disease, and immunosuppression. Patients with pre-existing skin lesion/infection, or infection in another site, and treatment with steroids and immunosuppressive drugs are more prone to get surgical wound infection due to impaired host defence mechanisms. These should be corrected or treated before an elective operation is planned.

Table 11.1 – Wound classification based on estimation of bacterial density, contamination and risk of subsequent infection.

Surgical procedure	Definition	Expected infection rate (%)
Clean	Nontraumatic, uninfected operative wounds in which no inflammation is encountered; there is no break in technique; and the respiratory, alimentary, or genitourinary tracts or the oropharyngeal cavities are not entered.	1 - 3
Clean-contaminated	Operation in which the respiratrory, alimentary or genitourinary tracts are entered under controlled conditions and without unusual contanmination.	8 - 10
Contaminated	Operation associated with: • Open, fresh trauma wounds • Major breaks in a sterile technique or gross spillage from the gastrointestinal tract • Acute, nonpurulment inflammation.	15 - 20
Dirty and infected	Operation involving old trauma wounds with retained devitalized tissue, foreign bodies, or faecal contamination, and those with existing infection.	25 - 40

Pre-operative hospitalization

Pre-operative stay in hospital should be kept to a minimum before operations because the longer the patient stays in the hospital before an operation, the greater becomes the likelihood of succeeding wound infection.

Pre-operative shaving

Pre-operative shaving is no longer recommended because shaving can cause small nicks and breaks leaving the skin bruised and traumatised which increases the risk of colonization and infection. If the hair must be removed, a depilatory cream may be used. Hair may also be clipped very short by using a clippers where necessary. If shaving is thought to be necessary, it should be done immediately before the procedure to reduce the risk of infection.

Antibiotic prophylaxis

A relevant antibiotic(s) should be given at the correct time, ie at induction of anaesthesia. It should not be given for more than 24 hours, preferably one or two doses according to local antibiotic policy. Antibiotic prophylaxis is indicated for dirty or contaminated operations. Prophylaxis is usually given for clean operations where an infection constitutes a catastrophe for the patient, eg insertion of joint and cardiac prostheses, caesarean section with prolonged rupture of membrane, etc.

OPERATIVE FACTORS

Surgical hand scrub

Although sterile gloves are worn for surgical procedures, the skin of the hands and forearms should be scrubbed (see page 160) to reduce the number of microorganisms from personnel to the patient. Surgical scrub not only removes debris and transient microorganisms from the nails, hands, and forearms but also reduces the resident microbial count to a minimum. Rings, watches and bracelets should be removed and fingernails should be kept short and clean. The hands and forearms should be free of open lesions and breaks in the skin.

Skin disinfection

It is essential that the operating site is well disinfected before incision. Apply 70% ethanol or 60% isopropanol, preferably with 0.5% chlorhexidine or 10% povidone iodine. This should be applied with friction well beyond the operation site for at least 3-4 minutes and allowed to dry. The use of antiseptic with alcohol increases the risk of burns to the patient during diathermy, especially if the alcohol is not allowed to dry and drapes are soaked with alcoholic disinfectant, therefore the area must be allowed to dry before operating. Alternatively 7.5% povidone iodine "Betadine" or 0.5% aqueous chlorhexidine may be used.

Theatre wear

Theatre gowns: To avoid transfer of pathogens into the operating suite, clothes intended for work in the suite should not be worn in patient care outside the suite. The operating team should wear sterile gowns at surgery.

Gloves: Using gloves during surgery serves two purposes; it protects the surgical team from contamination by blood and exudate from the patient and the patient from transfer of microorganisms from the surgeon's hands. Single-use sterile disposable gloves should be used. They should not be washed or disinfected and re-used.

Masks: High efficiency filter masks should be worn by all members of staff scrubbed and assisting at the operating table. Wearing of masks by other members of staff not assisting the operation is not necessary. A fresh mask must be worn for each operation and care must be taken when the mask is discarded.

Eye protection: Mask and protective eye wear or face shields should be worn during procedures that are likely to generate droplets of blood or body fluids to prevent exposure of mucus membranes of the mouth, nose and eyes.

Hair/beard cover: All members of staff entering the theatre must wear their hair in a neat style. Long hair should be tied in such a way that when the head is bent forward hair does not fall forward. Hair must be completely covered by a close fitting cap made up of synthetic material. Beards should be fully covered by a mask and a hood of the balaclava type which is tied securely at the neck.

Foot wear: Plastic overshoes are not necessary. If there is constant risk of spillage then ankle length antistatic boots should be worn.

Draping

To restrict the transfer of microorganisms to the wound and to protect the sterility of the instruments, equipment, supplies, and gloved hands of the personnel, a sterile field must be established by placing sterile drapes around the wound. The use of plastic incisional adhesive drapes is controversial and is not associated with a reduction in infection rate.

Wound drains

It is generally accepted that wound drains provide access for bacterial entry via colonization and hands. Drains should not be used as an alternative to good haemostasis. The closed system of wound drainage is indicated where drainage is essential. Open wound drains are not considered appropriate and may lead to an increase in wound infection.

Surgical technique

The skill of the surgeon has a central role in minimising surgical wound infection. Expeditious surgery, gentle handling of tissue, reduction of blood loss or haematoma formation, elimination of dead tissue, debridement of devitalized tissue, removal of all purulent material by irrigation or suction, and removal of all foreign materials from the wound are essential to minimise surgical wound infections in all patients.

Staff movement

Excessive presence and movement of staff contributes to an increase in air-borne bacterial particles. In the case of bacterial skin infections, dispersal of pathogens (*Staph. aureus*, β-haemolytic streptococci) may be large. It is advisable to keep operating theatre staff to the essential minimum. Additional personnel who wish to view the operation can be accommodated in the surgical viewing suites, where available. Staff with a boil or septic lesion of the skin or eczema colonized with *Staph.aureus* should not be allowed in theatre.

The door to the operating room should be closed at all times to avoid mixing corridor air with the operating room air, which would increase the number of the microorganisms.

Operating theatre ventilation

In the United Kingdom, the design and other operating parameters for a theatre system are set in various documents laid down in the Department of Health guidelines, codes and building notes (see references).

Conventionally ventilated theatre: To prevent contaminated air from reaching the operating theatre, mechanical ventilation is recommended. The air within the operating room should be at a positive pressure compared with other theatre suite rooms and with the external corridors. Theatre ventilation must be checked regularly and maintained by an appropriate engineer. Written records of all work on the ventilation system must be kept by the works and maintenance department. Coarse and fine air filters must be replaced regularly according to the manufacturer's instructions or when the pressure differential across the filter indicates that a change is required.

A minimum of 20 air changes per hour of filtered air should be delivered. The temperature of the room should be maintained between 15 to 25°C. The humidity should be maintained between 40 to 60% for staff comfort and to inhibit microbial growth. Additional ventilation units, such as mobile air cooling devices, must not be introduced into the theatre without consultation with the Infection Control Team.

The minimum standard for microbiological air counts for the operating room is 30 colony forming units (cfu)/m^3 when the theatre is empty, and less than 180 cfu/m^3 when in use. A conventionally ventilated theatre requires microbiological checks at commissioning, immediately after commissioning and at any major refurbishment, by the Infection Control Team. Routine bacteriological testing of operating room air is not necessary but may be useful when investigating an outbreak.

Ultra clean air theatre: It is now accepted that ultra clean air (<10 cfu/m^3) reduces the risk of infection in implant surgery. To achieve this, laminar flow systems (airflow 0.5 m/s) which deliver about 300 air changes per hour or special ventilation combined with bacteria impermeable clothing has to be used.

The operating parameters for an ultra clean air theatre are different from those for a conventionally ventilated theatre, and depend upon the design of the system. In a fully walled enclosure, the airflow 1m from the filter face should not fall below 0.3 m s^{-1}, but in a partially walled enclosure, because there is a greater diffusion of air, the airflow at 1 m from the floor (above the level of the operating table surface), should not be less than 0.2 m s^{-1}. Bacterial counts at 1 m from the floor should be less than 1.0 bcp m^{-3} (bacteria carrying particle) of air in an empty enclosure and when tested during an operation there should be less than 10 bcp m^{-3} at the level of the operating table at the centre of the enclosure. Additionally, if the system is partially walled, then on each of the four sides at the periphery of the enclosure the bacteriological count should not exceed 10 bcp m^{-3}.

Ultra clean air theatres require assessment not only at commissioning, but regular bacteriological assessment is mandatory as a part of routine service to the theatres, because factors other than simple ventilation parameters are important in determining the quality of the air. Ideally the microbiologically checks should be performed every three months, because of the long incubation period for joint sepsis and any system defect needs to be detected early and rectified quickly.

Duration of operation

There is a direct link between the length of the operation and the infection rate with clean wound rate, doubling every hour. This is because the bacterial contamination increases over time and the operative tissues are damaged by drying and other surgical manipulations, ie retractor, use of diathermy, etc.

Miscellaneous factors

1. All sterile packs should be opened using a technique that will prevent contamination of a sterile instruments.

2. All clinical waste should be disposed of according to the local policy.

3. Infected cases should preferably be last on the list.

4. Staff who are carriers/dispersers of *Staph.aureus* (including MRSA) and with septic lesions should seek advice from the Occupational Health Department and should not work in the theatre until the condition resolves.

5. Cleaning of the theatre should be carried out according to the written protocol.

POST-OPERATIVE FACTORS

Wound dressing

Staff should be trained in the appropriate method of dressing the wound. Frequency of dressing should be kept to a minimum and should not be opened for 48 hours after the operation, unless infection is suspected. The longer a wound is open, and the longer it is drained, the greater the risk of contamination.

Clean, undrained wounds seal within 48 hours and are unlikely to be infected in the ward. Ward-acquired infection is less common than intra-operative infection and is often superficial. On the other hand, theatre-acquired post-operative infections are usually deep-seated and often occur within 3 days of operation or before the first dressing. Many infections, particularly after prosthetic surgery, may not be recognised for weeks or months.

Post-operative stay

Avoid post-operative stay and overcrowding in the ward and discharge the patient as soon as possible. If this is necessary for medical reasons, keep the patient in a clean environment to protect from colonization with bacteria from infected patients.

Surveillance

Surveillance of wound infection is a useful tool to demonstrate the magnitude of the problem. This should be combined with a regular feedback to the surgeon. This exercise has shown to provide strong motivation and reduction in the infection rates in clinical practice. With quicker turn around time of the patients in hospital, ideally surveillance of wound infection should include follow up of all the patients in the community to ascertain the actual incidence of post-operative infection for which resources are required.

References and further reading

Cruse PJE, Foord R. The epidemiology of wound infections: a 10 year prospective study of 62,939 wounds. *Surgical Clinic of North America* 1980,**60**:27–40.

Horan TC, Gaynes RP, Martone WJ, *et al*. CDC definitions of surgical sites infections,1992: a modification of the CDC definitions of wound infections. *American Journal of Infection Control* 1992; **20**: 271-274.

Classen DC, Evans RS, Pestotnik SL *et al*. The timing of prophylactic administration of antibiotics and the risk of surgical-wound infection. *New England Journal of Medicine* 1992; **326**: 281-286.

Ayliffe GAJ. Role of environment of the operating suite in surgical wound infection. *Reviews of Infectious Diseases* 1991; **13**(Suppl 10): S800-804.

Department of Health. *Health Building Note 26; Operating Departments*. London: HMSO, 1991.

Department of Health and Social Services. *Ventilation of operation department. A design guide*. London: DHSS, 1983.

Holton J, Ridgway GL. Commissioning operating theatres. *Journal of Hospital Infection* 1993; **23:** 153-160.

Emmerson M. Environmental factors influencing infection. In: Taylor EW, ed. *Infection in Surgical Practice*. Oxford: Oxford University Press, 1992: 8-17.

Kluytmans J. Surgical Infections Including Burns. In: Wenzel RP, (ed). *Prevention and Control of Nosocomial Infections*. 3rd ed. Baltimore: Williams & Wilkins 1997: 841-865.

Roy MC. The Opening Theatre: A Special Environment Area. In: Wenzel RP, ed. *Prevention and Control of Nosocomial Infections*. 3rd ed. Baltimore: Williams & Wilkins 1997: 515-538.

12

HOSPITAL SUPPORT
SERVICES

KITCHEN, CATERING AND FOOD INSPECTION

The importance of adequate food hygiene facilities is paramount, since the consequence of an outbreak of food poisoning in a health care facility can be life threatening for patients whose immune system is compromised by their medical condition. Although catering staff are mainly responsible for providing food in hospitals, nursing and domestic staff are also involved in distributing or serving meals to the patients. Everyone who handles, prepares, processes and distributes food must understand the principles of basic food hygiene and good food-handling practices and should fully realise their own role in the prevention of food-borne illness. All food must comply with the Food Safety Act and the Food Hygiene Regulations (see references).

Inspection: The catering manager has responsibility for the catering services. Daily inspections of kitchens and all food handling areas is necessary by catering managers and supervisory staff with the aid of check lists. Health authorities/ Area Boards are responsible for food hygiene in hospitals. Full inspections should be carried out twice yearly by the hospital management, catering manager, the Consultant in Communicable Disease Control (CCDC), the Infection Control Doctor (ICD), Environmental Health Officer (EHO) and a member of the estates department. Full reports of these inspections should be submitted to the hospital Chief Executive and the hospital Infection Control Committee. A Code of Practice for EHOs states the minimum frequency of inspections, which is calculated using a risk assessment scheme. EHOs inspect food handling premises in accordance with the guidelines of their Institute, current legislation and approved code of practice and have statutory responsibilities and powers which extend to hospital premises.

Table 12.1 – The commonest causes of food poisoning

Preparing food too long in advance.

Storing food at ambient temperatures.

Cooling food too slowly before placing in refrigerator.

Not reheating food to temperatures at which food poisoning bacteria can be destroyed.

Using contaminated food.

Undercooking meat, meat products and poultry.

Not thawing frozen poultry and meat for long enough.

Cross contamination between raw and cooked food.

Keeping hot food below 63°C.

Infected food handlers.

Reproduced with permission from Barrie D. The provision of food and catering services in hospital. *J Hosp Infect* 1996; **33:** 13-33.

Food handlers: All food handlers should complete a pre-employment questionnaire, which is reviewed by a person competent to assess the implications of any positive answers and decide if examination of faecal specimens is necessary. Pre-employment stool testing is not generally required in the absence of a history of enteric fever.

All food handlers with infections, diarrhoea or suspected gastrointestinal infection **must** stop working and report to their manager. Return depends on whether it is considered safe, usually by the Occupational Health Department, but the opinion of the medical microbiologist/ICD or CCDC may be sought.

Ward kitchens: Ward kitchens or food-handling areas and staff using them should observe the same levels of food and personal hygiene as other food handlers. There should be specific written cleaning and waste disposal policies. The Infection Control Team with the CCDC and the local EHO should draw up codes of practice for food handling in ward kitchens.

Nurses should understand when and why extra precautions are indicated for patients with gastrointestinal infections, and be reminded that person-to-person spread of certain enteric pathogens (eg, *Salmonella* spp. *Shigella* spp. etc) infection is more common in maternity, paediatric, care of the elderly and psychiatric patients in whom faecal soiling is more likely.

Table 12.2

GENERAL RULES OF FOOD HYGIENE

Delivery	Accept frozen food below -18°C. Accept chilled food below +3°C. Check "within date" code. Check state of packaging.

Storage	Practise stock rotation.
	Provide clean, dry, pest-free conditions.
	Keep at correct temperatures.
	Keep covered until required.
	Keep raw foods separately from cooked items
	     – use separate utensils, surfaces,
	     – wash hands between different foods.

Thawing	Thaw below 15°C. Thaw completely. Cook with 24 hours.
Cooking	Ensure centre of food reaches 70°C for 2 minutes. Cook on the day of consumption or chill rapidly and refrigerate within 1½ hours. Consume within 3 days. Hold below 10°C or above 63°C.
Reheating	Avoid, if possible. Reheat rapidly. Attain 70°C (use temperature probe).
Distribution	Hot food above 63°C. Cold food below 10°C. Check with temperature probe.
Waste	Discard unwanted food after 1 hour. Always cover food waste.
Cleaning **Maintenance**	Observe schedules for all items. Ensure good state of service and repair.

Reproduced with permission from Barrie D. The provision of food and catering services in hospital. *J Hosp Infect* 1996; **33:** 13-33.

Ward refrigerators, dishwashers, microwave ovens and ice-making machines are used by nursing staff, domestic staff and visitors, and so are often used incorrectly. Ward kitchen refrigerators should be used solely for patients' food and never for medicines, units of blood, pathology specimens, etc. Ice-making machines should be purchased in consultation with the Infection Control Committee and planned maintenance and cleaning protocol should be drawn up by the ward manager as advised by the Infection Control Team.

Management of outbreaks: The hospital Infection Control Team should, in conjunction with the CCDC and EHO, draw up a detailed policy and procedures for use in the event of an outbreak of food-borne illness as part of a general outbreak plan (see chapter 1). These should include a list of names and on-call telephone numbers, so that appropriate persons can be contacted. The procedures should be discussed and endorsed by the hospital Infection Control Committee.

References and further reading

Department of Health and Social Security. *The Report of the Committee of Enquiry into an Outbreak of Food Poisoning at Stanley Royd Hospital.* London: HMSO, 1986.

Department of Health. *Chilled and Frozen. Guidelines on Cook-Chill and Cook-Freeze Catering systems.* London: HMSO, 1989.

Department of Health. *Management of outbreaks of foodborne illness.* London: Department of Health,1994.

Department of Health. *Food handlers: Fitness to work.* London: Department of Health,1995.

Department of Health and Social Security. *Health Service Catering Hygiene.* London: DHSS,1986.

Food Safety Act. London: HMSO, 1990.

Food Safety (General Food Hygiene) Regulations 1995 Food Hygiene (General) Regulations. London: HMSO,1995.

Department of Health. NHS Management Executive. *Management of Food Services and Food Hygiene in the National Health Service.* HSG(92)34, 1992.

Barrie D. The provision of food and catering services in hospital. *Journal of Hospital Infection* 1996; **33:** 13-33.

Department of Health. NHS Management Executive. *Hospital catering - delivery of a quality service.* EL (96)37, 1996.

LAUNDRY POLICY

Although soiled linen has been shown to be a source of large numbers of pathogenic microorganisms, the risk of actual disease transmission is negligible. Common sense, basic principles of infection control and accepted recommendations for handling and processing procedures must be adhered to minimise the risk of infection. These recommendations must be adhered to regardless of the use of in-house or off-site contract of laundry services to minimise the potential risk of hospital-acquired infection associated with soiled linen to staff handling and laundering linen. Management should ensure that all staff, and laundry contractors responsible for handling or laundering linen are appropriately trained. They should comply with the guidance laid down by the NHS Executive in the HSG(95)18; these should be incorporated into contracts where laundry services are not provided in-house. The following principals should be followed for safe handling of laundry:

- All personnel involved in collection, transport, sorting, and washing of soiled linens should be adequately trained, wear appropriate protective clothing and have access to hand washing facilities.

- Used linen must be put into the appropriate colour coded container as soon as possible after removal and must be handled with care at all times, as agitation of fabrics can markedly increase the number of airborne bacteria.

- Clean and soiled linen must be transported separately. Clean linen must be covered or wrapped for protection from contamination during transport. Protection of stored linen in a clean area of the ward or department is recommended until the linen is distributed for patient use.

- Soiled linen processing areas must be separated from clean linen storage, patient care areas, food preparation areas, and clean supply and equipment storage areas.

- Laundry bags should not be stored in wet places and must be protected during transport.

- On arrival in the laundry, infected linen should be handled only by the inner bag and placed directly into a designated machine and processed by thermal or other disinfection processes.

Inadvertent disposal of objects (sharps and personal property) in linen is a common problem. Therefore all staff are urged to remove these objects which not only endanger staff in the laundry from sharps injuries but these objects can cause extensive damage to expensive laundry machines. Theatre staff often leave tissues in the pockets of scrub suits which cause problems because they disintegrate into countless fragments during laundering and are deposited on main compartments which are very difficult to remove.

Categories of linen

Used linen: Over 90% of the hospital linen falls into this category. *Used linen* (soiled and fouled) covers all used linen irrespective of state, apart from that which is designated as infected linen. *Soiled linen* is used linen which requires laundering but is neither fouled nor infected, while fouled linen is used linen which is contaminated with excretions, secretions, blood or body fluids. In some geriatric and psychiatric units up to 80% of the linen is classified as fouled linen. For transportation, such linen should be placed into polythene or nylon/polyester laundry bags. All bags must be securely fastened before being sent to the laundry. Handling policy for used (soiled and fouled) linen will be determined at the local level with the advice from the Infection Control Committee.

Infected linen: used linen which has been used for a patient with known or suspected infections, ie gastroenteritis (*Salmonella* spp., *Shigella* spp. etc), patients with infectious hepatitis, AIDS/HIV infection, open pulmonary tuberculosis, notifiable diseases and other infections caused by microorganisms in hazard group 3 (refer to the ACDP guidelines). *Infested linen* should be dealt with as infected linen. Linen from a patient with hazard group 4 microorganisms (refer to the ACDP guidelines) must be steam-sterilized by autoclaving within the group 4 containment unit before laundering. To reduce the risk of infection to hospital and laundry staff, infected linen is placed immediately into a bag which is water soluble or has a water soluble membrane. The bag is closed in an outer red plastic bag. At the laundry the outer bag is removed and the closed inner bag is transferred to a designated washer extractor. All infected linen should be labelled as to its origin.

Heat-labile linen: Fabrics damaged by the normal heat disinfection process and likely to be damaged at thermal disinfection temperatures. They are normally laundered in wash extractors at temperature of 40°C, and dried at 60°C. Therefore, their use by patients infected with hazard group 3 microorganisms should be avoided whenever possible. Fabrics must be checked before purchasing to ensure that they will withstand the relevant laundering processes.

Colour coding of laundry bags

Used linen (Soiled and fouled): Soiled linen should be put into white fabric bags. Fouled linen should be first put into a clear white (or off-white plastic) bag and then placed into a white fabric bag.

Infected linen: Double bag using an inner water soluble bag (or bag with water soluble membrane) and then put into a red plastic bag (or red colour should be a prominent feature on a white or off-white background). Additionally, it should carry a prominent yellow label marked "Infected Linen".

Heat-labile linen: Should be put into a white bag with a prominent orange stripe.

References and further reading

NHS Executive. HSG (95)18. *Hospital laundry arrangements for used and infected linen.* London: 1995.

Advisory Committee on Dangerous Pathogens (ACDP). *Categorisation of biological agents according to hazard and categories of containment.* 4th ed. London: HMSO, 1995.

Barrie D. How hospital linen and laundry services are provided. *Journal of Hospital Infection* 1994; **27:** 219-239.

DISPOSAL OF CLINICAL WASTE

Under the requirement of the Health & Safety at Work Act 1974, and to comply with the Environment Protection Act, associated regulations, and a clearly defined waste management strategy are required. Failure to comply with these requirements could lead to legal penalties which, in the event of an incident, may include criminal proceedings against individuals. Chief Executives and general managers have a duty under the Health & Safety Act 1974 and COSHH regulations (1988) to demonstrate that they are providing a safe working environment. They should ensure that responsibility is delegated to a responsible person to implement of the acts and the regulations, and ensure implementation is monitored and their written health and safety policies reflect the requirement of the regulations. Each member of staff must ensure that they are aware of and abide by the requirements of that policy.

Health and Safety commission gives the following scheme for categorisation of waste:

1. ***Clinical Waste:*** Clinical waste is categorized into following groups:

   Group A: All human tissue, including blood (whether infected or not), animal carcasses and tissue from veterinary centres, hospitals or laboratories, and all related swabs and dressings. Soiled surgical dressings, swabs and other soiled waste from treatment areas and waste materials, where the assessment indicates a risk to staff handling them, for example from infectious disease cases.

   Group B: Discarded syringe needles, cartridges, broken glass and any other contaminated disposable sharp instruments or items.

   Group C: Microbiological cultures and potentially infected waste from pathology departments (laboratory and post-mortem rooms) and other clinical or research laboratories.

   Group D: Certain pharmaceutical products and chemical wastes.

   Group E: Items used to dispose of urine, faeces and other bodily secretions or excretions assessed as not falling within Group A. This includes used disposable bed pans or bed pan liners, incontinence pads, stoma bags and urine containers.

2. ***Non-clinical:*** Non-clinical or household waste is defined as other waste not in the categories of clinical waste or special waste. It is non-toxic, non-infectious or its basic nature is unlikely to prove a health hazard or give offence in its produced form.

3. ***Special waste:*** Special waste is defined as waste which is dangerous to life and difficult to dispose of by its nature, which is further classified into Pharmaceutical, Cytotoxic and Radioactive. It is beyond the scope of this book to give details and readers are advised to refer to the local policy.

Specification of clinical waste bags

Clinical waste bags should be:

- of a maximum nominal capacity of $0.1m^3$.
- be of minimum gauge of 225 (55 microns) if of low density, or minimum gauge 100 (25 microns) if of high density.
- match the chosen container or fittings in use.
- be coloured yellow, the standard colour (BS No. 309).

Plastic bags when used in high risk areas (ie, laboratory, infectious disease and isolation units) and disposal of human tissue should be of a minimum gauge 800 (200 microns) if of low density, or minimum gauge of 400 (100 microns) if of high density. Purpose-made plastic ties should be used for sealing these bags.

Table 12.3 – Types of waste containers and final disposal.

Colour of Bag	Type of Waste	Final Disposal
Yellow Bag (Colour BS 309)	All waste (ie, clinical waste) destined for incineration.	Incineration
Light blue or transparent with light blue inscription (Autoclave bag). (Colour BS 175)	Waste for autoclaving (eg, in laboratories) or equivalent treatment before ultimate disposal. This bag must be put into yellow plastic bag (ie, double bagged).	Incineration
Yellow sharps box (BS 3720)	For disposal of used sharps.	Incineration
Black plastic bag (Colour BS 381C)	Normal household waste: not to be used to store or transport clinical waste.	Landfill
Black/white cardboard box	For aerosols, broken glass, glass bottles etc.	Landfill

Methods for safe handling and disposal of clinical waste

The plastic bags should be secured in a foot operated lidded bin or carrier frame. The lid will bear a label denoting the category of waste and the appropriate colour of bag.

- The bags are sealed when three-quarters full. Lighter weight bags may be secured by tying the neck, while heavy duty bags require a purpose made plastic tie or closure. Staples **must not** be used, as they may cause a sharps injury to the handler.

- The bags should be identified by tying a label with the name of the health care facility or hospital and the department concerned, which clearly identifies the point of origin, or by closing the bag with pre-printed coded bag clips issued by the hospital responsible for the final disposal by incineration. Pre-printed coded bag clips issued to a particular health care facility or department should not be used by another department as the code on the clip is individualised for each department.

- Heavy duty protective clothing should always be worn when handling waste bags. The bags should be handled by neck only and kept upright. To avoid injuries, do not put your other hand underneath the waste bag while lifting.

- Waste is stored in a neat fashion within a designated collection area of each ward or department, which must be secured against unauthorized access and must be removed from clinical areas daily or more frequently if necessary. The area should be cleaned when necessary and kept dry. Central collection or storage points must be secured from unauthorized access, elements, pests or rodents.

- Blood and body fluids which are contained in a secure container, eg enclosed suction systems such as a receptacle, etc, must be carefully handled and transported to final disposal by incineration. Waste from non-disposable apparatus, ie suction bottles etc, must be poured gently into a sluice hopper and flushed away.

- Bulk transport vehicles are the responsibility of the transport manager. Loaded vehicles leaving the health care facility or hospital site must be properly secured. Should spillage occur, this must be dealt with safely. The vehicle must have a regular cleaning and disinfection schedule.

- Household waste is disposed of by landfill and may be compacted. Clinical waste must not be compacted prior to disposal. Human tissue, (ie limbs) must be enclosed in a heavy duty double yellow plastic bag and disposed of by incineration under supervision. Placentae must be placed into an appropriate container and must be disposed of as clinical waste by incineration.

- All employees who are required to handle and move clinical waste should be adequately trained in safe procedures and in dealing with spillages or other incidents for their area of work. A record of training should be kept.

- Staff who regularly have to handle, transfer, transport or incinerate clinical waste containers must be provided with appropriate protective equipment, ie heavy duty gloves, appropriate footwear, and industrial apron or leg shields, waterproof clothing, a face visor or respiratory equipment as required.

- Spillages should be treated according to the methods outlined in the disinfection policy.

- All accidents and incidents involving clinical waste, particularly those resulting in injury to or contamination of handlers, must be reported without delay to the line manager who should:

  - record and report the accident through the normal accident reporting system.

  - initiate first aid and containment of the spillage without delay, as required by the circumstances of the incident.

  - refer the injured staff to the Occupational Health Department or Accident & Emergency department as appropriate, according to the local policy.

  - report the incident to a member of the Infection Control Team for assessment, investigation and advice if required.

References and further reading

NHS Executive. *Health Guidance Note. Safe disposal of clinical waste whole hospital policy guidance*. London: HMSO, 1995.

London Waste Regulation Authority. *Guidelines for the segregation, handling, transport and disposal of clinical waste*. 2nd ed. LWRA, 1994.

Health and Safety Commission. *The safe disposal of clinical waste*. London: HMSO, 1992.

Department of the Environment, Scottish and Welsh Office. *Waste management: The duty of care, a code of practice*. London: HMSO, 1992.

Collins CH, Kennedy DA. *The Treatment and Disposal of Clinical Waste*. Leeds: H and H Scientific Consultants Ltd, 1993.

SAFE USE, HANDLING AND DISPOSAL OF SHARPS

Sharps are any items that can cause laceration or puncture wounds. Examples include discarded hypodermic needles, instruments used in invasive procedures (eg blood-sampling, surgery, dentistry, acupuncture, ear-piercing and tattooing); emergency services' cutting equipment, broken glass and jagged metal. General principles for handling and use of sharps are:

– Avoid sharps usage wherever possible.

– Never leave sharps lying around; dispose of them carefully.

– Do not keep syringes, needles or any other sharps object in your pocket.

– Used needles must not be resheathed unless there is a safe means available for doing so.

– Do not use needles if there is any suspicion for example a broken seal, that they may have been used previously.

Methods of safe disposal of sharps

• It is the *personal responsibility* of the person using a sharp to dispose of it safely as soon as possible after use. Where the specific clinical procedure prevents the user from doing this, the user still retains overall responsibility for safe disposal of sharps.

• If a sharp has been accidentally dropped, it must be recovered and disposed of properly. If the search is unsuccessful, the individual should ensure that other people using the area are informed so that they can take care. It is particularly important to notify cleaning staff of the possible danger. The person-in-charge of the area should be notified and a record kept, until the sharp has been found and properly disposed of.

• Needles and syringes should be discarded as a single unit, where this is possible, into a designated sharp box.

• Glass slides, glass drug ampoules, razors, disposable scissors and IV cannulae must be discarded into a sharps box.

• The attached sharps from IV blood/solution administration sets must be cut off with scissors and discarded into the sharps box. The used scissors must be cleaned properly using an alcohol impregnated wipe.

• Scalpel blades should be removed using a surgical blade remover and then discarded into a sharps box. Non-disposable sharps should be placed in a suitable secure container to await decontamination.

- After blood has been collected, and to avoid haemolysis, the needle may require removal from the syringe before transfer of blood into the collection tube. The needle should be removed from the syringe and discarded into a sharps box.

- When syringes containing arterial blood are to be sent to the laboratory, needles **must** be removed and the nozzles of the syringes sealed by means of a luer rubber cap or a blunt hub.

- Health care workers must not re-use the barrel (needle holder) of vacuum blood collection systems ("vacutainer") where there is visible blood contamination or where blood has been taken from a patient who is known or suspected to be infected with a blood-borne virus.

- When an injury occurs with a contaminated sharp, bleeding should be encouraged and the site should be washed under running water (see page 154). The injured member of staff should immediately report the incident to their line manager who should then refer them to the Occupational Health Department or, out-of-hours, to the local Accident and Emergency department according to local policy. The injured person should complete an Accident Report form with full details of the injury for investigation and action by the local Infection Control Nurse, to minimise its recurrence.

Use of sharps boxes

- All sharps boxes must be correctly assembled and used according to the manufacturer's instructions. They should conform to British Standard 3720 and be kept in a location which excludes injury to patients, visitors and staff.

- They should be readily available wherever blood samples are taken. The person-in-charge of the ward or department is responsible for ensuring safe handling and disposal of sharps within their own area.

- Sharps containers should be closed securely when three-quarters full and placed at a designated secure collection point. The sharps container **must** never be overfilled since used sharps protruding from overloaded containers constitute a very significant hazard to those who have to handle them. The lid of the sharps box must not be used as a means of ensuring that the needle and syringe 'fit' inside the box.

- The used sharps boxes must be suitably marked for identification from wards or departments of the hospital or the health care facility. This enables the exact location and responsibility for any offending container to be determined.

- Do not use sharps boxes for any other purpose ie storage of ward items, etc.

- In the ward, sharps boxes must be securely stored whilst awaiting collection. Pottering and transport staff must take special care and should wear heavy duty gloves when collecting sharps containers.

References and further reading

British Medical Association. *The Safe Use and Disposal of Sharps*. London: BMA, 1993.

Gwyther J. Sharps disposal containers and their use. *Journal of Hospital Infection* 1990; **15:** 287-294.

Collins CH, Kennedy DA. Microbiological hazards of occupational needlestick and "sharps" injuries. *Journal of Applied Bacteriology* 1987; **62:** 385-402.

INDEX

D

Q

Q fever, 41

Quaternary ammonium
compounds, 60, 62

R

Rabies, 41

Radioactive waste, 195

Razors, 78

Resident microorganisms, 157

Respiratory isolation precauions
body fluid spills, 25
CSSD, 25
decontamination & waste
disposal, 25
equipment, 25
hand hygiene, 25
inter-departmental visits, 25
laboratory specimens, 25
last offices, 25
laundry, 25
location, 24
protectitive clothing, 24
staff, 24
visitors, 24

Rhino/laryngscope, 78

Rifampicin, 39, 92

Ringworm, 41

Rubella, 36

S

Salmonella spp. (Salmonellosis), 41

Scabies, 42

Schistosomiasis, 42

Scissors, 79

Sharp injury, 17, 152-155, 198
exposure and prophylaxis against
HIV, 155
immediate contact procedure, 154

management of sharp injury, 152,
153
prophylaxis against hepatitis B
infection, 153

Sharps, 16, 199-200
safe disposal, 199, 200
safe use, 199, 200
sharp boxes, 200

Shaving brushes, 79

Sheepskins, 79

Shigellosis spp, 40

Shingles, 37

Soap, 79, 161

Sodium dichlorocyanurate
(NaDCC), 56

Spillages
blood and body fluids, 70

Spirometry, 178

Sputum container, 79

Staff health , 17, 147-155
immunization against
hepatitis B, 151
needle-stick/sharps injury, 152-155
post-exposure management after
contact with tuberculosis, 149-151
pre-employment health
questionnaire, 148
protection against
tuberculosis, 149-250

Staphylococcal infection
food poisoning, 42
See also MRSA

Sterilization , 52

Streptococcal(β haemolytic)
infection, 42

Strict isolation, 20
body fluid spills, 22, 70
decontamination & waste
disposal, 22
equipment, 22
hand hygiene, 22
inter-departmental visits, 23
laboratory specimens, 23
last offices, 23
laundry, 22